GORGEOUS FOOD
gluten free

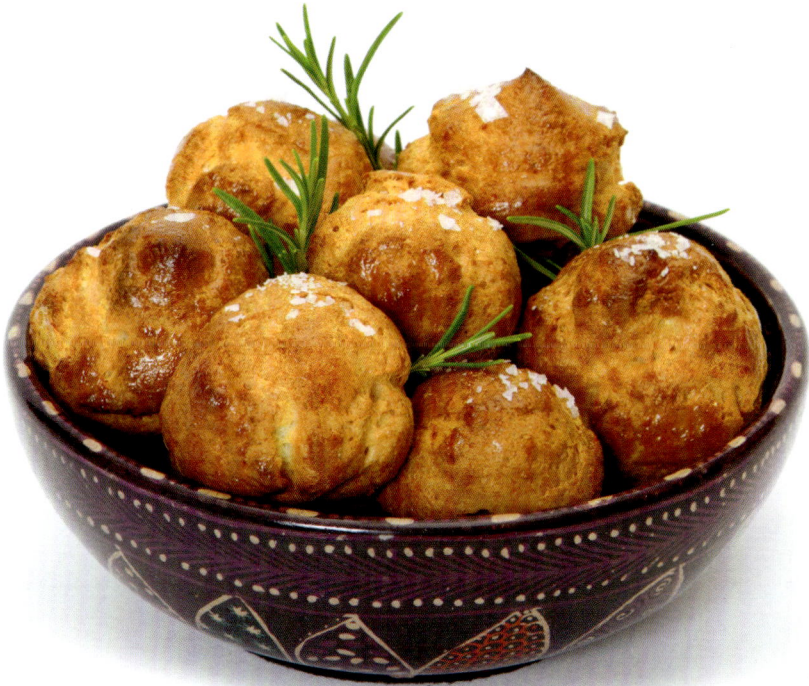

Venetia Blackman

WP

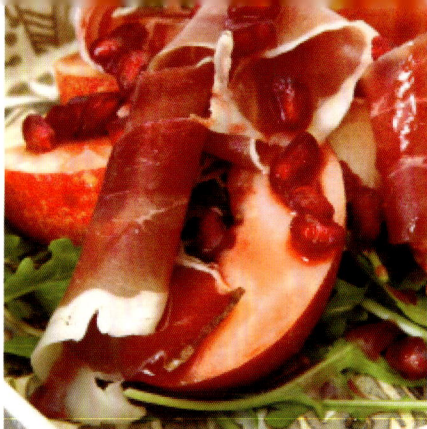

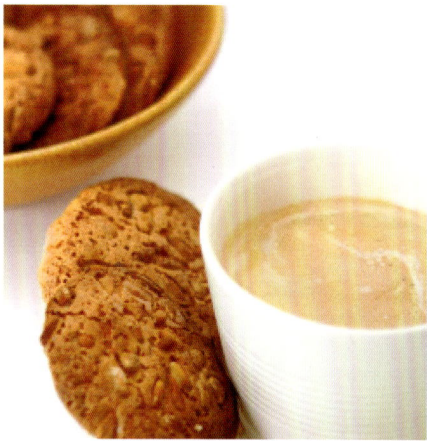

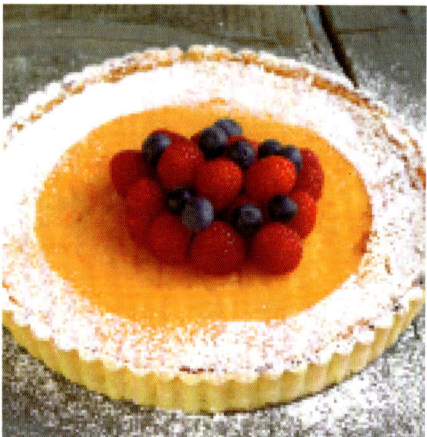

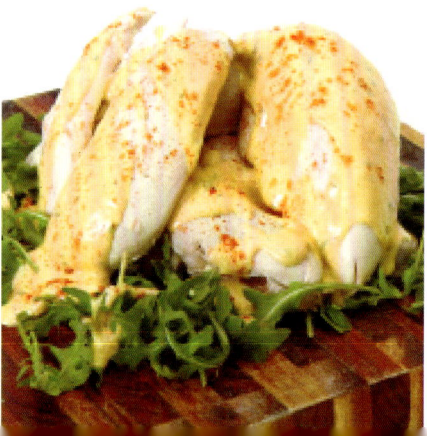

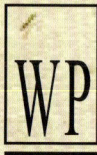

Published by:
Wilkinson Publishing Pty Ltd
ACN 006 042 173
Level 4, 2 Collins St Melbourne,
Victoria, Australia 3000
Ph: +61 3 9654 5446
www.wilkinsonpublishing.com.au

International distribution by Pineapple Media Limited
(www.pineapple-media.com)   ISSN 2203-2770

National Library of Australia Cataloguing-in-Publication entry

Author: Blackman, Venetia, author.

Title: Gorgeous food gluten free / Venetia Blackman.

ISBN: 9781922178411 (paperback)

Subjects: Gluten-free diet--Recipes.
Gluten-free foods.

Dewey Number: 641.56318

Layout Design: Tango Media Pty Ltd
Cover Design: Tango Media Pty Ltd

Photos by agreement with Rod Stewart.

Venetia was born in Melbourne as the second youngest of five. She had a typical upbringing in the western suburbs of Sydney as well as regional towns in both New South Wales and Victoria. She has called Melbourne home since 2001, where she lives with her husband Jeremy and two dogs: Lucie and Bon-Bon (Bonnie).

Venetia has enjoyed cooking since she was a child and considers herself to be a high caliber home cook. She is a self-confessed Francophile with a strong French and broader European influence evident throughout her recipes.

Venetia works for the Australian Public Service and during her career has been fortunate to have had the opportunity to work on and lead programs and initiatives to enhance the services provided to the Australian community.

This is her first book.

"We all know someone who cannot eat gluten. We know others who are simply trying to reduce the amount of gluten they and their families consume. I have written this book to give everyone the opportunity to prepare beautiful and delicious food that just happens to be gluten free."

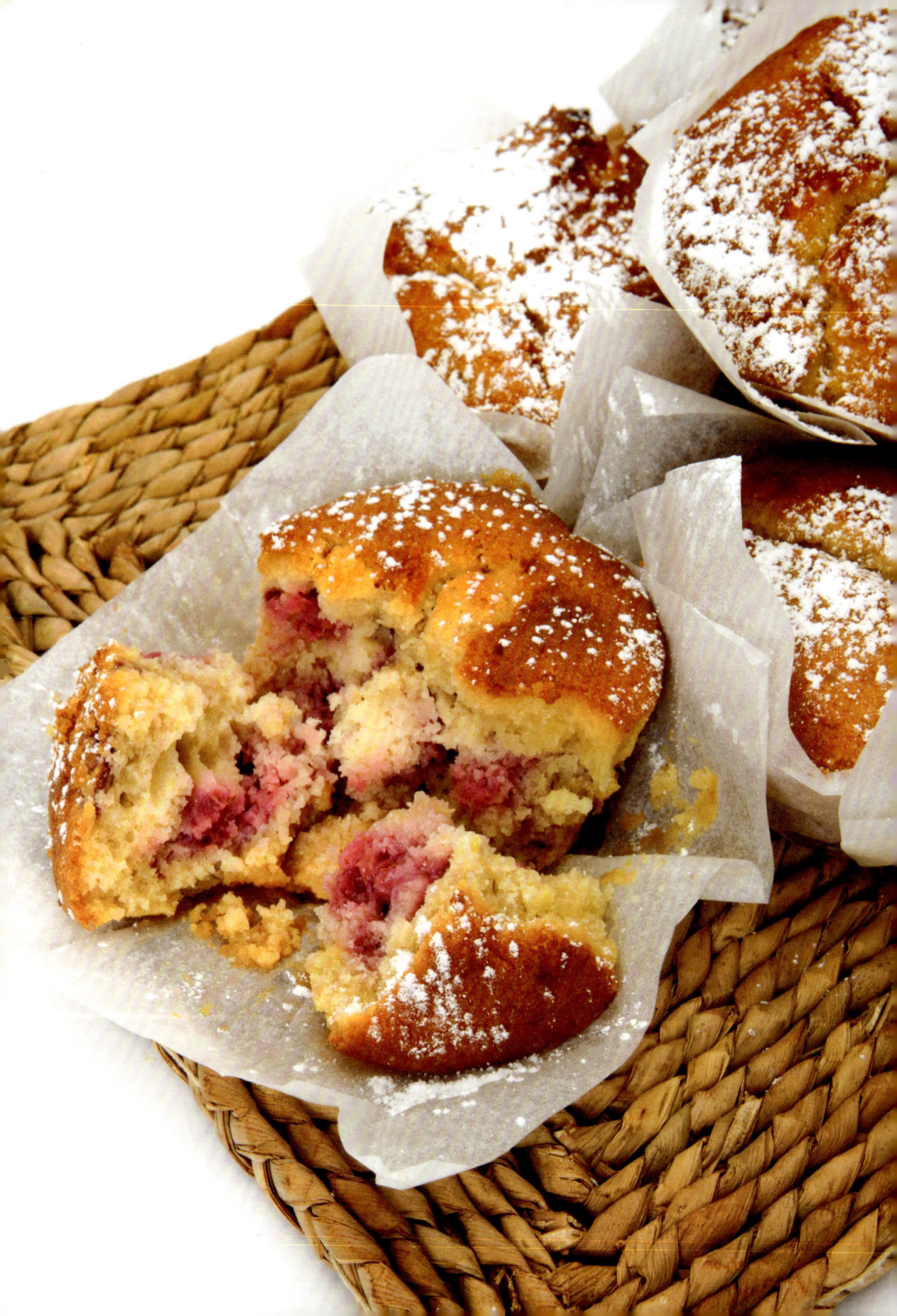

Contents

introduction

I WAS DIAGNOSED with Coeliac disease at eighteen months of age, which means that I have lived, laughed and loved while maintaining a gluten free diet since before I can remember.

Common opinion would suggest that I have eaten sub-par food all my life because 'gluten free' and 'delicious' are generally considered to be mutually exclusive. I'm glad to say that my experiences have been far from disappointing. Beautiful food (that just happens to be gluten free) has been a big part of each and every day.

My fondest childhood memories take place in my mother's kitchen. It was a large room with, what seemed to my young eyes, an enormous table in the centre of it. The table filled the space and its wooden top had been scrubbed clean so many times over the years that the edges were the only place the varnish had managed to survive.

I used to sit at that table each evening while I did my homework. My mother would be preparing dinner for me and my four siblings at one end of the table and I would sit about half-way along, on the side furthest away from the stove, so as not to get in her way. We would talk about my day while she peeled potatoes and oscillated between the chopping board and whatever pot was on the stove. When dinner was ready I would clear away my books and set the table before we all sat down to eat.

My mother certainly taught me how to cook the usual things children learn: chocolate cakes, cookies, anything sweet. However I don't believe that my cooking stems from these lessons but rather through a sort of osmosis. Watching someone cook who has finely tuned taste buds allows you to absorb information in much the same way as the flavours of a marinade permeate a piece of meat. You learn how flavours combine, what browning meat actually looks like, the smell of brandy as it hits a pan of buttery shallots. But most of all, you take in everyday things like how to chop an onion and the importance of always tasting, tasting, tasting. I still recall moments such as my mother and I checking the ripeness of pineapples - the sweet tangy smell at the base and how easily one of the centre leaves can be removed from the top.

Now, don't misunderstand me, I have eaten my fair share of truly awful food — who hasn't? Back in the early 80s gluten free products were difficult to find and in many cases were economically prohibitive.

If you did sink your life savings into the purchase of a packet of pasta, the resulting sludge in the bottom of the pan was your reward.

How wonderful it is today then, to be able to walk into any supermarket and purchase a packet of gluten free pasta that can be successfully cooked till al dente; that when served at a dinner party with a lovely marinara sauce is accompanied by ooo's and ahh's and exclamations of gratitude and appreciation. What a shame that so many of the gluten free pastas sold today still leave you with that pan of sludge. Why do they remain? Is it because so many people are convinced that gluten free food won't taste as good as 'normal' food? Or is it that continuing belief that if it tastes terrible, or the texture is compromised, it must be because there's no other way to make it gluten free? From discussions with so many people over the years this does seem to be the prevailing sentiment.

Through these experiences I have sought to find and create food that provides happiness and pleasure to those people that share their lives with me. The exclusion of gluten in these moments has not diminished our enjoyment but rather it has fuelled my desire to provide food that does not compromise on the integrity of my ingredients, or the satisfaction of my guests.

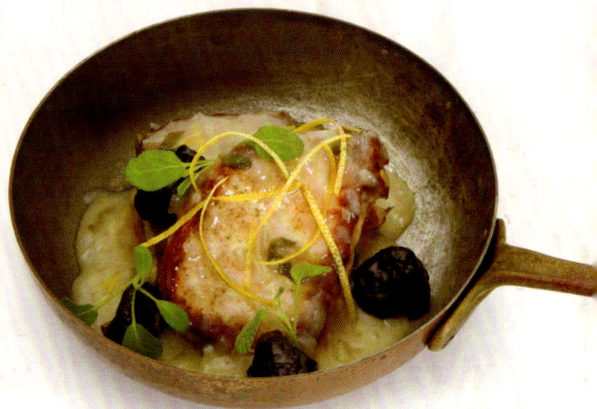

I'm so glad the intervening 25 years since I sat at that kitchen table doing my homework have been spent experimenting and learning about flavours, textures and how best to utilise what were often foreign ingredients to create my dishes — dishes in which the flavours, textures and presentation are never compromised, but rather augmented through the process of their development. Through it all has been my aim of creating truly great food that just happens to be gluten free.

This book is full of recipes that have resulted from my explorations and I hope they bring you and your loved ones as much joy and happiness as they have to me and mine.

why gluten free?

AS SOMEONE diagnosed with Coeliac disease, I and around one in every one hundred people must maintain a gluten free diet to survive. It's generally recognised that a further 14 people in that hundred have an intolerance to wheat and another 15 people in that hundred choose to modify their gluten consumption in some way.

The concept of 'gluten free' has become well-known across the community and most people now have some awareness of what it means to maintain a gluten free diet. When I speak with people about gluten free and ask them if they know much about it, I usually hear a response along the lines of: *"So that means you can't eat bread and pasta and that sort of thing, yeah?"*

I have on occasion had people ask me if I have to maintain a gluten free diet, citing friends who seem to avoid it sometimes but then on other occasions will happily enjoy eating a custard Danish.

When holding these conversations I often ask the person to describe their food consumption on a typical day. Here is one such overview: a bowl of cereal for breakfast; a couple of biscuits with cheese for morning tea; a salad sandwich for lunch; a muffin for afternoon tea; and pasta for dinner.

I then explain that every single meal they described contains gluten in multiple forms and, on almost every occasion, the gluten derived from wheat. I then ask them if they were to have potato salad at lunch time would they be likely to have some mashed or baked potatoes with their dinner. Of course the answer to this question for most people would be "No"; we have all been educated about the need to eat a balanced diet.

So why do we think it's ok to eat a sandwich for lunch and some pasta for dinner? Because gluten disguises itself in so many forms of food, from the obvious such as bread and pasta to the more obscure such as the mayonnaise on your sandwich and the jar of pre-prepared pasta sauce.

It is for this reason that so many people are choosing to reduce their gluten consumption — to achieve a truly balanced diet. Many people also find that a move to a diet containing less gluten comes with health and wellness benefits such as feeling less bloated and sluggish.

I'm not an advocate for people maintaining gluten free diets if they don't have a medical condition that requires it but I do wholeheartedly believe that all people should try to reduce the amount of gluten they are consuming so that they achieve more balance in their diet and also as a preventative measure against the future development of a gluten-related disorder.

Gluten free cookbooks often focus on the dietary aspect of their ingredients and the nutritional benefits of the dishes. While this approach is admirable, it often makes for average or even boring results.

My recipes are designed for home-cooks at varying levels of skill in the kitchen, to create amazing food with beautiful flavours and textures that 'just happen to be gluten free'. If the dish isn't as good as or better than a recipe containing gluten, then more work is needed before the recipe is ready to be served. This way we don't have to compromise on flavour or texture and the recipes can be enjoyed by everyone — gluten *and* gluten free eaters.

Many people also find that a move to a diet containing less gluten comes with health and wellness benefits such as feeling less bloated and sluggish.

ingredients

MOST OF THE ingredients I use are unprocessed or base ingredients - I like to know exactly what is in the food I am eating. This has an added benefit in that I'm not buying pre-packaged and pre-prepared food, which in my experience tends to create less-than-excellent results and is still relatively expensive.

The only specialist gluten free products I buy on a regular basis are bread and pasta. Now, there are many products on the market with a full array of quality on offer from the absolutely terrible (to the point that on occasion I ask myself how they even made it to market) through to the truly exceptional and everything in between.

Here are a few of my learnings from over the years:

Pasta

When buying gluten free pasta I find the best results come from those that use a blend of both rice and maize. There are a few brands on the market with my current picks being:

✳ San Remo range: a good all-rounder which is available from most supermarkets.

✳ Schar: the best gluten free pasta range I have found thus far. It's not as widely available but a good health food store will be able to order it in for you. It is imported from Italy and is sold in almost every pharmacy and health food store across Europe.

My husband and I use the Schar pasta as it has a beautiful texture and is successfully cooked to al dente. Jeremy finds in much easier to digest than gluten pasta and it leaves him feeling lighter and less bloated.

Bread

It is extremely difficult to produce
a quality gluten free loaf. The gluten
found in wheat flour is what creates the
lovely chewy texture of a good slow risen
sourdough or country loaf.

There are other options though
and flat breads are a good alternative
with a range of brands popping up on
supermarket shelves in recent times.

For a quality bread that is similar
in texture and flavour to rye bread I
recommend the Schar 'Pane-casereccio'.
I use this for fresh or toasted sandwiches
and it is absolutely perfect for bruschetta.
Schar has a wide range of breads including
a beautiful brioche, which they sell as
'Bon Matin', and are great heated in a low
oven and then eaten with slightly salted
butter and homemade jam.

recipe list

Breakfasts

Buckwheat pancakes with fresh cherries
Creamy scrambled eggs with parsley
Grilled peaches with yoghurt and almonds
Corn fritters with avocado salsa
Potato rosti with smoked salmon
Raspberry and white chocolate muffins
Egg and bacon pies
Crêpes with lemon and sugar

Sweet Things

Lemon and yoghurt syrup cake
Fudgy chocolate brownies
Peanut butter cookies
Banana and pecan cupcakes
Marmalade and polenta cookies
Pikelets
Fresh summer plum cake
Corsican macarons

Lunches

Corn and avocado salsa
Green bean, artichoke and avocado salad
Bruschetta of sardines, oranges and fennel
Poached chicken with mango mayonnaise
Potato salad
Caprese salad
Nectarine, roquette and proscuitto salad
    with raspberry vinaigrette
Apple, fennel, onion and roquette slaw

Savoury Things

Cheesy corn and herb muffins
Gougeres
Pumpkin scones
Quail egg bites with bacon and chives
Onion jam tartlets with goat's cheese
Mini lamb meatballs with pinenuts
    and currants
Cucumber bites with smoked salmon
Cannellini bean dip with crudites

Entrees

Cream of chestnut soup
Crêpes with a creamy mushroom filling
Tarragon scallops wrapped in prosciutto
    with celeriac puree
Venetian inspired soup
Artichokes with lemon scented butter
Lamb fillets with pickled cucumber salad
Apple, grape, avocado and prawn jellies
Salad of orange with olives and fennel

Main Courses

Roasted pumpkin, spinach and
    pinenut lasagne
Perch with a caper, lemon and
    white wine sauce
Spaghetti with meatballs in tomato sauce
Whole baked trout with lemon and thyme
Beef and ale pie
Oven baked ratatouille
Braised pork chops with lemon and prunes
Tarragon roasted chicken marylands
    with gravy

Side Dishes

Green beans with toasted almonds
Cornbread
Ginger and orange carrots
Cauliflower and cheesy Swiss chard
Sautéed beetroot leaves
Braised cannellini beans
Pan-fried zucchini with garlic, mint
    and chilli
Warm puy lentils with shallot vinaigrette

Desserts

Apricot and sauvignon blanc jellies
Steamed golden syrup pudding
Chocolate fondants
Chocolate roulade filled with cream
    and fresh berries
Lemon tart
Spiced pear struesel cake
Saffron and vanilla poached pears
Caramel baked rice pudding

Breakfasts

GROWING UP in a household of five children, we saw breakfast as nothing more than the first fuel stop of the day. It was nutritious, filling and predictable — a bowl of cereal or maybe a piece of fruit and some yoghurt. Each person grabbed their own meal and staggered through the morning chaos of getting ready for school: music practice, feeding the guinea pigs, cats, dogs … fresh mulberry leaves for the silk worms in their shoe box. Then the last-minute panic of preparing lunch: assembling sandwiches, scrambling for a clean container and the final, full-on rush to reach the bus-stop in time.

Breakfast did become a much more inviting experience however, when Jim came to stay.

My childhood memory of Jim is of a six-foot-four brawny tank of a man with a mop of red hair and a face of beard. He had a deep booming Alaskan-accented voice, was quick with a jibe, and had a full-bodied, bellowing laugh. Jim is one of those characters who appear in your life for only a short time. He stayed with my family over summer for about three consecutive years when I was in my early teens.

Jim owned a gold mine in Alaska and during the harsh winter the permafrost makes mining an impossible activity so he would come out to Australia for our summer. Towards the end of each visit, Jim would prepare an Alaskan breakfast for us all. Now, as far as I could tell, the Alaskan breakfast is much like the cooked breakfasts found right across America with the only difference being that Jim's portion sizes relegated his countrymen's efforts to the welter-weight division – even for a nation renowned for super-sized everything!

Jim would head-off to shop the day before and return with enough ingredients to feed my entire family five times over. A 10 kilogram (22 pounds) bag of potatoes, 4 dozen eggs, 2 kilograms (4.4 pounds) of bacon, 5 kilograms (11 pounds) of tomatoes, 10 kilograms (22 pounds) of oranges and 4 litres (1 gallon) of milk. These, together with five bottles of the most exquisite maple syrup and pre-mixed dry ingredients for hotcakes, which he brought from Alaska, were the basis of our feast.

The following morning would find him in the kitchen grating potatoes for hash browns, mixing batter for the hotcakes, frying eggs and bacon rashers, cutting tomatoes and sprinkling them with dried oregano before placing them under the grill to soften and caramelise, juicing oranges and generally creating an epicentre of gastronomy in our kitchen. No-one was allowed to help, so it was best to make a swift exit and jump on a bike to help build up an appetite that in no way could ever meet the supply of food that would be waiting upon our return.

Jim would bellow when he was ready for us to invade the dining room and we would discover the table heaped high with steaming platters of delicious, heart-stopping, fried heaven. Jim would still be in the kitchen preparing more and more batches of hotcakes, bacon and eggs to ensure a ready supply of hot food.

We would commence eating. And after a good innings we would look at the table and fail to identify where we had made an impact. By this stage Jim had taken his seat and was probably onto his second plate, wearing a huge grin, and his beard glistening with syrup and bacon fat.

For one person to prepare food in these quantities, the end result (while full of love and flavour) was most certainly not of the most refined quality. But its bold and brazen sensibilities made for such colourful and joyful memories that whenever I reflect on these moments I feel a smile spread across my face.

While the scale of these moments may not be something I have desired to replicate, in my adult life I have sought to create breakfast moments of this same joie de vivre and generosity of spirit. The recipes in this chapter have provided just this to friends and family, and formed the basis of new traditions which we carry forward and reflect on with the same feelings of joy and contentment.

Buckwheat pancakes with fresh cherries

It's Sunday morning and a couple of friends are staying for the weekend. This is the perfect thing for breakfast. It's special enough to show you care, and simple enough to pull together while recovering from the mischief of the night before. The salty bacon coupled with the slightly bitter & earthy buckwheat are perfectly complemented by the sweet maple syrup and fresh burst of cherries.

200 grams (1¼ cups) of buckwheat flour

60 grams (½ cup) of glutinous rice flour

5 grams (1 teaspoon) of gluten free baking powder

10 grams (2 teaspoons) of golden caster sugar

A pinch of salt

4 eggs

500mL (2 cups) of buttermilk

36 cherries stoned and halved (if you can't get fresh cherries try blueberries or tinned cherries)

8 rashers of bacon

Maple syrup

1. Turn your oven on, set it to a temperature of 120°C/250°F and place a plate covered with a kitchen towel on the bottom self.

2. Place the buckwheat flour, glutinous rice flour, baking powder, golden caster sugar and salt in a bowl and stir to combine.

3. Separate the eggs, placing the whites in the bowl of your mixer and combine the yolks with the buttermilk in a smaller bowl. Add the buttermilk and egg yolk mixture to the flour and mix lightly until just combined.

4. Whisk the egg whites until stiff peaks form and using a large metal spoon, fold the egg whites through the buckwheat batter in two batches ensuring they are well combined while maintaining as much air in the batter as possible.

5. Heat a large frying pan over a medium heat and brush a small amount of melted butter over the base. For each pancake, ladle approximately 4 tablespoons of batter into the pan and scatter with 6 cherry halves. Cook for about 2 minutes, or until bubbles appear on the surface of the pancakes then turn them over and cook for another minute. Transfer to the plate in the oven to keep warm while you make the remaining pancakes.

6. Once you have made all the pancakes (you should have 12) and they are keeping warm in the oven, cut the bacon rashers in half and fry till the desired level of crispiness is achieved.

7. To serve, place three pancakes on each plate in a lovely tall stack. Top with crispy bacon and drizzle with maple syrup. Eat while piping hot and make sure you have some extra maple syrup on the table.

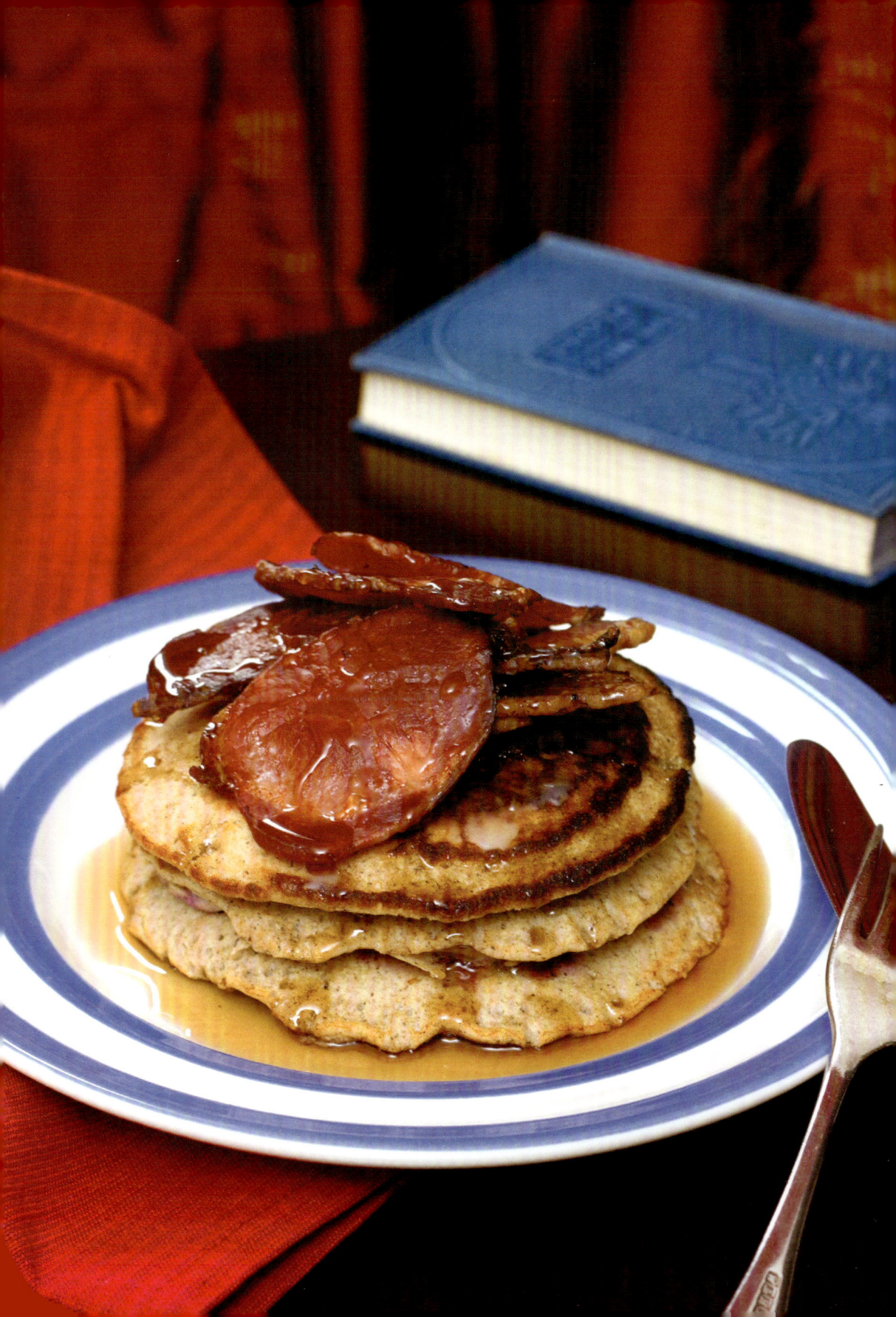

Creamy scrambled eggs with parsley

— SERVES 2 —

The perfect scrambled eggs should be creamy and velvety – they are so simple to make but rarely found. This is how I like to make them but experiment to find your own perfection.

6 eggs

80mL (4 tablespoons) of thickened (heavy) cream

¼ cup (small handful) of finely chopped parsley

Salt and pepper

Knob of butter

Hot buttered toast

1. Crack your eggs into a medium sized bowl, add the cream and parsley and season with salt and pepper to taste. Whisk until all the ingredients are well incorporated. Make sure you get the toast on so it's ready the moment your eggs are done.

2. Place a small saucepan on a medium heat and add a knob of butter. Once the butter is melted and foaming pour the egg mixture into the saucepan. Stir the eggs continuously with a wooden spoon ensuring you keep pulling the mixture away from the edges and scraping the bottom to maintain an even texture. The key is to continue to stir the eggs until they reach your desired consistency.

3. As soon as they are ready place them on the hot buttered toast and serve immediately. Delicious!

It is always a tough decision as to how to prepare the eggs for a Sunday morning brunch. Soft-boiled, poached, fried, scrambled...so many choices. But ultimately the perfect creamy scramble wins out more often than not. Delicious!

Grilled peaches with yoghurt and almonds

— SERVES 2 —

I adore white peaches as I find their flavour to be a little sweeter and their texture a little more refined. When they are in season, I simply cannot resist their scent. I hesitate to guess how many kilograms I must purchase over each summer and consequently this treat is a regular Sunday breakfast for my husband and me.

4 slightly firm white peaches

40 grams (2 tablespoons) of light muscovado sugar

80 grams (4 tablespoons) of thick Greek-style yoghurt

40 grams (2 tablespoons) of slivered almonds

1. Place a small frying pan over a medium heat and once warmed scatter the almond slivers over the base. Keep moving the almonds around the pan as their natural oils are slowly released and the nuts turn a beautiful golden brown. Please don't be tempted to leave them in the pan as they don't take long to toast and, if not constantly moving, have a tendency to burn. As soon as they have reached the desired colour tip them into a small bowl and set them aside while you prepare the rest of the dish.

2. Turn on your griller at a medium setting to heat up while you prepare the peaches. Cut the peaches in half and remove the stone from each. Place a griddle pan on a medium heat and once warmed place the peach halves into the pan with the cut side facing upwards. Let the peaches cook for a couple of minutes so their bottoms soften slightly and colour a little.

3. Take the peaches off the heat and scatter half a tablespoon of sugar over the cut surface of each before placing the griddle pan under the griller to allow the sugar to caramelise. This will take a few minutes as you want to ensure all the sugar crystals dissolve and mix with the juice that will be oozing from the peaches, which will in turn create a lovely golden toffee crust.

4. Once your peaches are ready remove the pan from the grill and place the peach halves on the serving plates. Spoon dollops of yoghurt on top of the fruit, scatter with the toasted almonds and serve immediately.

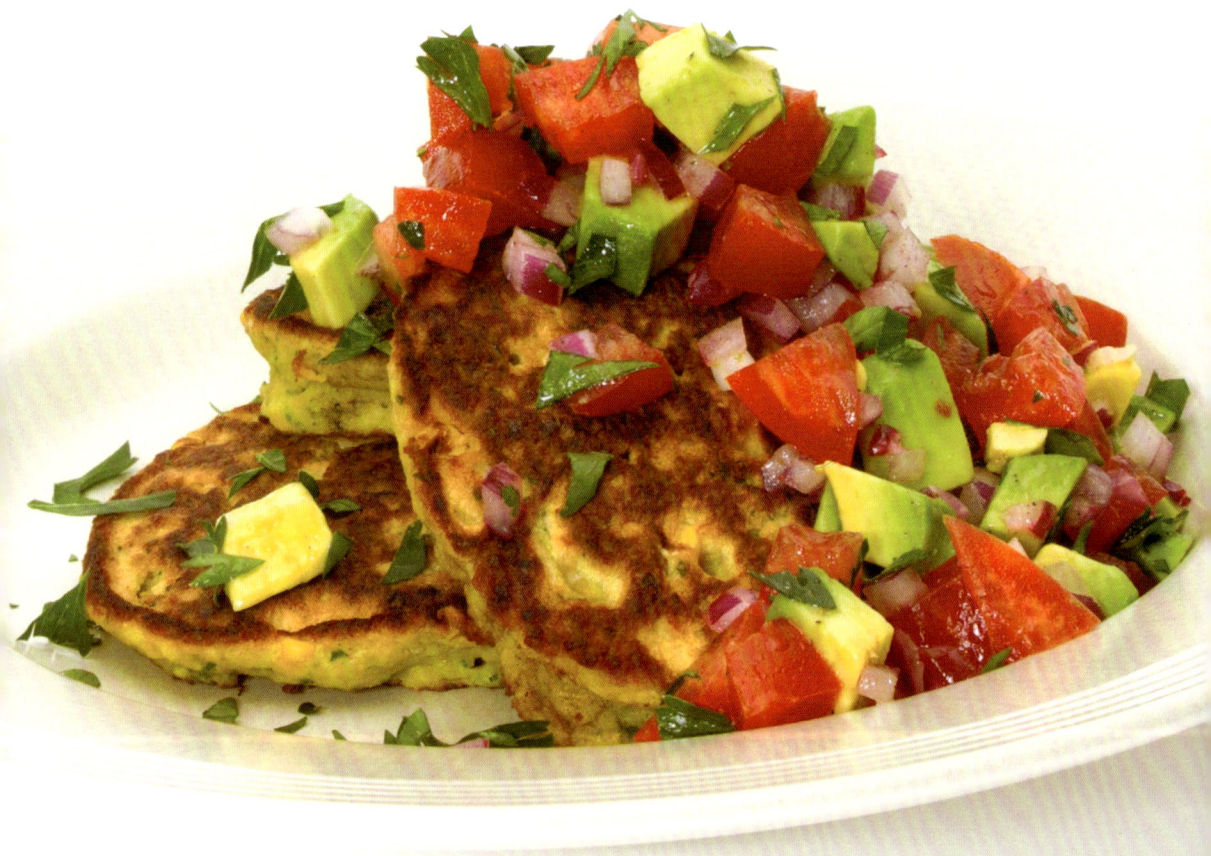

Corn fritters with avocado salsa

— SERVES.4 —

The blending of fresh corn kernels into the batter creates a beautifully moist result while the parsley turns the batter a wonderful forest green. The creaminess of the avocados slightly emulsifies the salsa, which brings all the flavours together. If you like a little bit of a kick, try adding a few splashes of Tabasco to the salsa.

FRITTERS

3 large corn cobs

1 small Spanish (red) onion

½ cup (large handful) of chopped parsley

2 eggs

95 grams (⅔ cup) of super-fine white rice flour

35 grams (⅓ cup) of glutinous rice flour

10 grams (2 teaspoons) of gluten free baking powder

Salt and pepper

Vegetable oil, for frying

AVOCADO SALSA

2 ripe avocados, stoned, peeled and diced

½ cup (large handful) of chopped parsley

40mL (2 tablespoons) of lemon juice

½ small Spanish (red) onion, finely chopped

1 tomato, seeded and finely chopped

Salt and pepper

Olive oil

1. Turn your oven on, set it to a temperature of 120°C/250°F and place a plate covered with a sheet of kitchen (greaseproof/baking) paper on the bottom self.

2. Pull the husks from the corn cobs and remove as much of the silk as possible. To remove the kernels from the corn cob, stand it on its end on your chopping board then with a sharp knife cut downwards between the core and the kernels. Repeat this process all the way around each of the cobs.

3. Place the kernels from two of the cobs and the onion, eggs, parsley, flours, baking powder, salt and pepper in a food processor and process until combined. Pour into a large bowl, add the remaining whole corn kernels and stir to combine.

4. Heat 1 tablespoon of the vegetable oil in a large frying pan over a medium heat. When the oil is hot, drop 2 heaped tablespoons of mixture per sweet corn fritter into the pan and cook in batches of 3 for 1 to 2 minutes on each side.

5. Drain on paper towels and keep warm in the oven while you are making the rest of the fritters. You should have enough mixture for 12 fritters. Serve with the avocado salsa.

6. If you can't get fresh corn you can substitute frozen kernels (about 500 grams) – just leave them to defrost before you start preparing the dish.

AVOCADO SALSA

Place all the ingredients in a bowl and stir very gently to combine. Season to taste and add enough olive oil to make the salsa glisten. Pile on top of the piping hot stacked sweet corn fritters and serve immediately.

Potato rösti
with smoked salmon

— SERVES 4 —

This dish is beautiful as a Sunday brunch sitting outside on a warm Spring morning. The combination of the horseradish in the crème fraiche coupled with the goat's cheese creates a sumptuous accompaniment to the fresh crisp cress and rich salmon. The golden rösti finishes off the dish with a lovely saltiness and crisp texture.

RÖSTI

4 désirée potatoes, peeled

2 eggs, lightly whisked

35 grams (¼ cup) of super-fine white rice flour

2.5 grams (½ teaspoon) of gluten free baking powder

20mL (1 tablespoon) of milk

Salt and pepper

Olive oil, to grease the pan

FOR PLATING

125mL (½ cup) of crème fraiche

2 teaspoons of horseradish cream

Juice of ½ a lemon

150 grams (5.3 ounces) of watercress or baby spinach leaves

16 slices (about 300 grams) of smoked salmon

100 grams (3.5 ounces) of fresh goat's cheese

Chives for garnish

1. Turn your oven onto a temperature of 120°C/250°F and place a plate covered with a sheet of kitchen (greaseproof/baking) on the bottom self.

2. Coarsely grate the potatoes, place them in a colander and rinse under cold running water. Drain them well and place on a dry tea (dish) towel. Bundle the towel up and squeeze out all the excess moisture.

3. Place the dry potato into a medium mixing bowl and add the eggs, flour, baking powder, milk and salt and pepper. Stir with a fork until the ingredients are well combined.

4. Heat a large non-stick frying pan over a medium-high heat and add a little olive oil. Using a large metal spoon, add a quarter of the potato mixture at a time to the hot pan and spread it out.

5. Cook the rösti for about 3 to 5 minutes until golden and cooked through. Turn over and cook the other side for about the same amount of time. Remove from the pan and place on some paper towel while you cook the other three rösti in the same manner.

6. Once you've made the rösti place one in the centre of each of your serving plates. Place the watercress in a mound in the middle of each rösti and then place the smoked salmon around the plate making the presentation as appetising as possible.

7. In a small bowl combine the crème fraiche, horseradish cream and lemon juice together and then drizzle over the salmon and cress. Crumble the goat's cheese over the top and finish with a few snips of the chives.

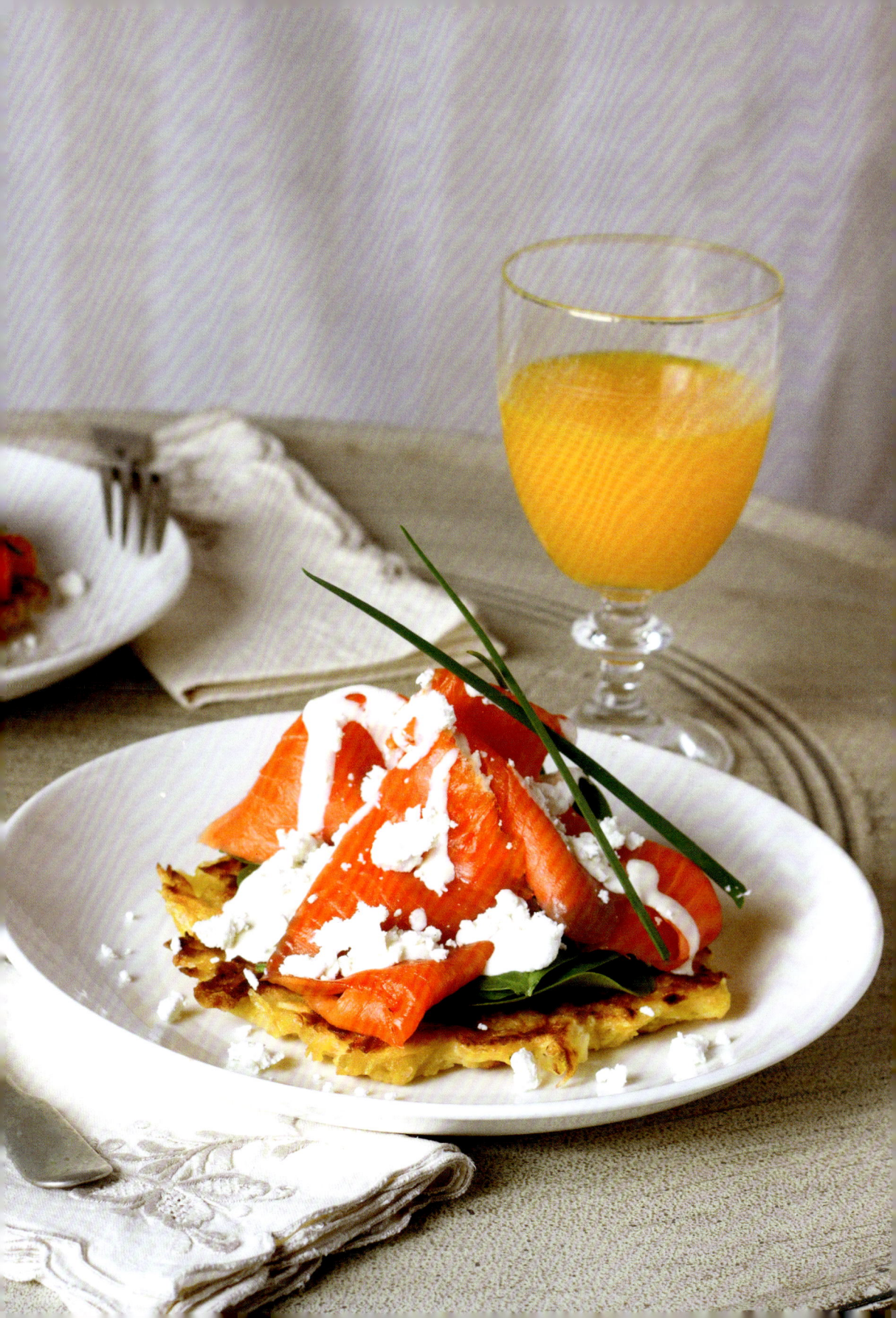

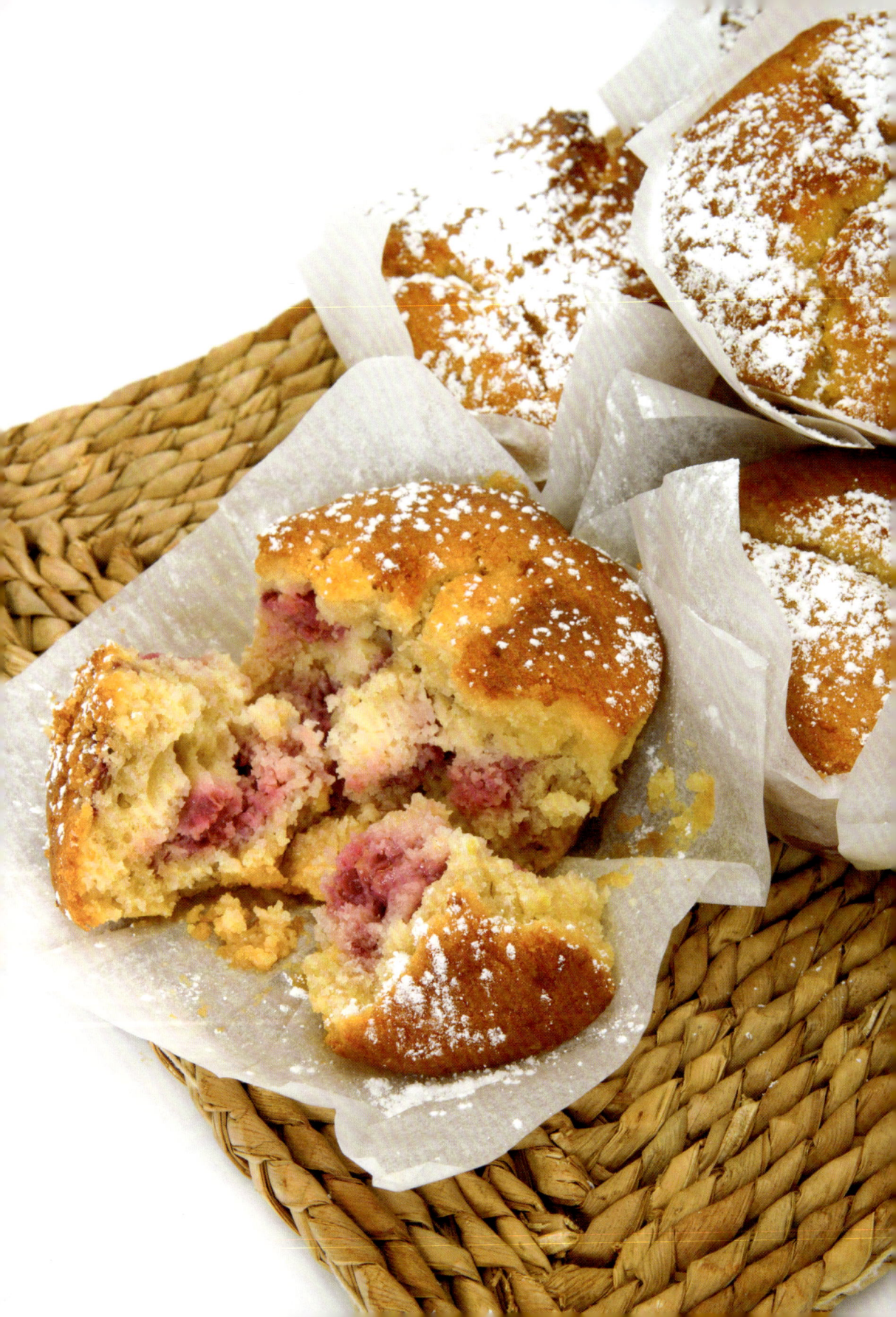

Raspberry and white chocolate muffins

— MAKES 12 —

Sometimes you just want something sweet for breakfast. To have something already prepared that you can grab as you run out the door, and hopefully make it to the train station in time, makes these muffins the perfect mid-week breakfast treat.

175 (1¼ cups) grams of super-fine white rice flour

90 grams (⅔ cup) of glutinous rice flour

15 grams (3 tablespoons) of gluten free baking powder

160 grams (¾ cup) of golden caster sugar

240 grams (8.5 ounces) of sour cream

2 eggs

Zest of one lemon, finely grated

85 grams (4½ tablespoons) of melted butter

225 grams (8 ounces) of fresh or frozen raspberries

175 grams (6 ounces) of chopped white chocolate

1. Place a shelf in the middle of your oven before preheating to a temperature of 180°C/355°F. Line your muffin tray with a piece of non-stick baking paper in each mould and ensure the paper is about half to 1cm (¼-½ inch) above the rim.

2. Into a medium sized mixing bowl sift the flours and baking powder and then add the sugar and stir to combine.

3. In a separate bowl combine the sour cream, eggs, butter and lemon zest with a balloon whisk. Gently fold through the flour and sugar mixture until combined.

4. Fold through the raspberries and white chocolate pieces and then spoon the mixture into the muffin moulds.

5. Bake for around 30 minutes or until a skewer comes out clean when inserted into the middle of a muffin. Let the muffins cool before dusting with icing sugar and serving.

My husband often comments that he doesn't like muffins, usually adding a reference to them being dry. These are nothing of the kind with beautiful fresh bursts of raspberry and molten white chocolate contributing to a moist and beautiful crumb.

Egg and bacon pies

— MAKES 8 —

I often make these pies for a weekend breakfast. My husband is a keen golfer and these make the perfect meal on the go. He will usually eat one before he leaves the house and then take one with him to munch on after the 'front nine'. They are lovely to eat at room temperature or straight from the refrigerator.

PASTRY

200 grams (7 ounces) of butter

165 grams (1¼ cups) of super-fine white rice flour

85 grams (⅔ cup) of glutinous rice flour

125mL (½ cup) of sour cream

FILLING

6 rashers of thickly sliced bacon

2 tablespoons of finely chopped parsley

1 tablespoon of finely snipped chives

9 eggs

Salt and pepper

1. Place a shelf in the middle of your oven before preheating to a temperature of 180°C/355°F. Grease the moulds of a muffin tray and set it aside while you prepare the pastry.

2. Into the bowl of an electric mixer add the butter and sifted flours. On a low speed mix until combined, increasing the speed as the mixture starts to come together. Add the sour cream and again mix to combine, starting slowly and increasing speed as the dough stabilises.

3. Roll out two-thirds of the dough to a thickness of about 3 millimetres (⅛ inch) and then cut out eight circles, each one large enough to cover the bottom and sides of your muffin tin. Place the pastry circles into the muffin tin moulds and shape them accordingly. The pastry is quite a soft dough so if you tear it or make a hole you should be able to easily fill it in with a little extra pastry.

4. Cut the bacon into lardons and lightly fry in a medium frying pan. Place them on some kitchen towel to drain any excess fat before scattering two thirds of the pieces into the pie shells. Scatter half the herbs over the bacon in the pie shells and then crack an egg into each, being careful not to break the yolks. Scatter the remaining herbs and bacon lardons over the top and then season with a little salt and pepper. Remember that the bacon will bring salt to the dish so be sure not to over season.

5. Roll out the remaining pastry dough and cut out eight circles, just larger than the top of your muffin tin moulds.

6. Whisk the remaining egg with a pinch of salt and brush over the edges of the pastry circles. Cover the pies with a pastry lid and then trim and seal the edges carefully. Brush the tops of the pies with the egg wash before placing them in the oven for around 25 minutes until they are rich golden brown. Allow the pies to cool to room temperature before removing them from the tin.

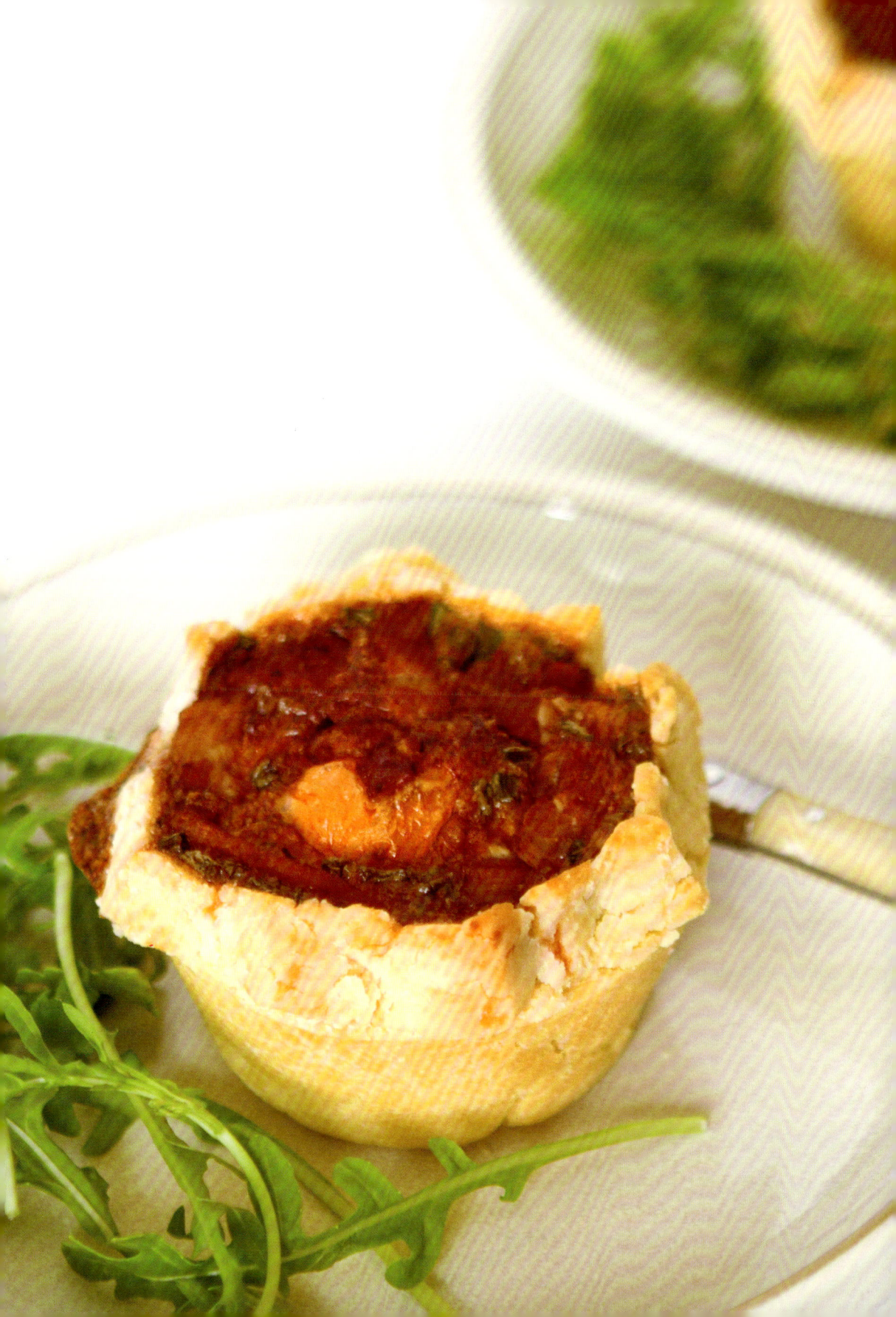

Crêpes with lemon and sugar

— MAKES 12 —

Crêpes are so versatile, you can have them with whatever fillings you like but my personal favourite is the simplicity of a sprinkling of golden caster sugar followed by a drizzle of freshly squeezed lemon juice.

3 large egg yolks

375mL (1½ cups) of milk

95 grams (⅔ cup) of super-fine white rice flour

35 grams (⅓ cup) of glutinous rice flour

20 grams (1 tablespoon) of golden caster sugar

60mL (3 tablespoons) of liqueur such as Grand Marnier or Brandy

100mL (5 tablespoons) of melted butter

Extra melted butter for the pan

Extra golden caster sugar for serving

Juice of two lemons

1. Turn your oven on to a temperature of 120°C/250°F and place a plate covered with a sheet of kitchen (greaseproof/baking) paper on the bottom self.

2. Sift the flours into a medium mixing bowl, add the sugar and stir to combine. Make a well in the centre of the flour and sugar mixture and add the egg yolks, milk and liqueur. Using a balloon whisk combine the ingredients until they form a smooth batter. Add the melted butter and whisk again to combine. The consistency of the batter should be similar to that of thickened cream.

3. Heat your crêpe pan over a medium to high heat and brush with a little of the extra melted butter. With a ladle place enough batter into the pan to form a delicately thin crêpe. I tend to pour the batter onto one side of the pan and as I pour I start to tip and swirl the pan so that the bottom of the pan is covered in a consistently thin layer.

4. Let the crêpe cook for a minute or two until the bottom is a lovely golden colour and then use an egg flip to turn and cook the other side for another minute.

5. Place the crêpe on the plate in the oven and remember to brush the pan with a little melted butter before you add the batter for the next crêpe.

6. Once you've made all the crêpes remove them from the oven and place them on the serving plates. Sprinkle them with golden caster sugar, drizzle with lemon juice and enjoy!

Sweet Things

I ALWAYS CRINGE when I hear someone say that the most important ingredient in any dish is love. Not because I disagree with them, but because I'm never sure if they really understand what that commonly used phrase means. Is it that you need to have love in your heart when you prepare the dish? Well this may certainly help, but unless this love translates into the act of preparing and cooking the dish, all the love in the world won't make that soufflé rise or that pork rind blister and crackle.

My less romantic (and pragmatic) interpretation is that you need to care about each step in the process and respect the ingredients by preparing them to the best of your ability. It's not about being clever or even a particularly gifted cook; it's just about being patient and taking your time. When a recipe says "a finely chopped onion" then an extra couple of minutes to ensure that the result is a fine chop rather than a rough chop will make all the difference to the end product. In a recipe there might be ten little things like this that need to be done, and if each one of them is done well and with care you have given yourself the best chance of creating a plate of perfection at the end.

Baking is one area of cooking where those "little things" can be the difference between a lovely fluffy sponge cake and a rubber mat at the bottom of your cake-tin.

I love to bake, and I think this is in part due to the fact that as a cook you are truly in touch with, and in control of, each step in the process. Many people are scared of baking — it's too precise...too many measurements... I'm not so sure... Yes the measurements matter, but you can be just as creative as you are when concocting a new salad. The ratio of vinegar to oil in a vinaigrette is just as important as the ratio of egg to flour in a sponge cake.

Many gluten free baking recipes use a range of flours and gums to try to create a 'gluten-like' product, and while some of these are successful, I find them unnecessarily complicated and often compromised in terms of flavour or texture. In this chapter I have tried to keep things simple but delicious, with the main focus being on traditional processes and concepts.

Lemon and yoghurt syrup cake

— SERVES 12 —

The tartness of lemon coupled with the slightly astringent yoghurt balances out the sweetness of sugar and makes for a lovely light and exciting cake. This is one of my favourites to make if friends are coming for afternoon tea. It is best accompanied by a dollop of luscious cream on the side.

100 grams (3.5 ounces) of unsalted butter, softened

150 grams (⅔ cup) of golden caster sugar

2 eggs

160 grams (5.6 ounces) of natural yoghurt

Zest and juice of a lemon

115 grams (⅔ cup plus 2 tablespoons) of super-fine white rice flour

60 grams (⅓ cup plus 1 tablespoon) of glutinous rice flour

15 grams (3 teaspoons) of gluten free baking powder

1. Place a shelf in the middle of your oven before preheating to a temperature of 170°C/340°F. Grease a 23cm (9 inch) spring-form cake tin with butter and then line the base with grease-proof paper.

2. Place the softened butter and two-thirds of the sugar into the bowl of your bench-top mixer. With the whisk attachment secured, start at a low speed to roughly incorporate the ingredients before turning to the highest speed setting and allowing it to beat until the mixture is white and fluffy. You may need to stop the mixer occasionally to scrape down the sides.

3. If you don't have a bench-top mixer then you can cream these ingredients by hand with a wooden spoon or with a pair of hand-held rotary beaters.

4. You can check if the mixture is ready by rubbing a small amount between your thumb and forefinger — you shouldn't be able to feel the sugar crystals anymore as they will have dissolved.

5. Once the mixture is ready, add the eggs one at a time, beating until each is completely incorporated and the mixture has returned to its fluffy texture.

6. Add the yoghurt and lemon zest and beat until incorporated and the mixture is smooth.

7. Place a sieve over the mixing bowl and sift in the rice flours and baking powder. Gently fold through the dry ingredients with a large metal spoon until combined and then spoon the mixture into the cake tin and smooth the surface.

8. Place the cake in the pre-heated oven and bake for around 30 minutes. You can check if the cake is cooked by placing a wooden skewer into the centre and if it comes out clean then it is ready. It will also have just started to pull away from the sides of the tin.

9. Once you have removed the cake from the oven you can prepare the syrup. Combine the lemon juice and remaining 50 grams of sugar in a small saucepan and place it over medium heat while stirring until the sugar dissolves. Bring the syrup to a boil for around 1 to 2 minutes or until it just thickens slightly.

10. Pour the hot syrup over the now warm cake and leave it to cool in the tin before serving.

Fudgy chocolate brownies

The lovely earthy crunch of the walnuts and the sweet sticky prunes make for some textural interest as you eat these lusciously fudgy brownies. Eat them as they are or top them with some vanilla bean ice-cream for a truly decadent dessert.

185 grams (6.5 ounces) of dark chocolate

125 grams (½ cup) of unsalted butter

115 grams (⅔ cup) of dark muscovado sugar

2 eggs

95 grams (⅔ cup) of super-fine white rice flour

45 grams (⅓ cup) of glutinous rice flour

170 grams (6 ounces) of pitted prunes, roughly chopped

100 grams (3.5 ounces) of walnuts, roughly chopped

1. Place a shelf in the middle of your oven before preheating to a temperature of 175°C/345°F. Grease and line a 20cm (8 inch) square cake tin and set it aside while you prepare the brownie mixture.

2. Place the butter and chocolate into a medium saucepan and over a moderate heat stir continuously until it melts and combines. Remove the saucepan from the heat and set it aside to cool before adding the sugar and eggs. Using a wooden spoon beat the mixture immediately to ensure the eggs are well incorporated into the melted chocolate and butter.

3. Sift the flours into the saucepan and fold them through the chocolate mixture. Beat the mixture for about 2 minutes before adding the prunes and walnuts and folding them through.

4. Pour the mixture into the waiting cake tin and place in the pre-heated oven to bake for around 25 minutes. You will know the brownies are ready when they are still soft in the centre but no longer wobble when touched.

5. Remove the tin from the oven and leave the brownies to cool in the tin before cutting them into squares and serving.

Peanut butter cookies

— MAKES 24 —

I think these cookies were probably the first thing I ever baked. I'm not sure where the original recipe came from but over the years I've played with it by adding all sorts of different things. Children and adults alike love the crunchy and chewy texture of what must be one of the simplest recipes in the world.

400 gram (14 ounce) tin of sweetened condensed milk

250 grams (1 cup) of smooth peanut butter

90 grams (3 cups) of cornflakes

1. Place a shelf in the middle of your oven before preheating to a temperature of 175°C/345°F. Add the condensed milk and peanut butter to a medium sized mixing bowl and stir with a wooden spoon until well combined. Roughly crush the cornflakes in your hands as you add them to the bowl. Give everything a good mix to ensure each flake is coated in the sticky gooey mixture.

2. Use a teaspoon to scoop out the mixture and roll it between your hands to make small balls. Place the cookie balls onto a baking tray leaving space around them to spread. This recipe makes approximately 24 cookies so 2 standard sized baking trays will be sufficient. Once you've rolled all the balls, licked your fingers and then washed your hands thoroughly use the back of a teaspoon to push down on the top of each ball so you end up with little rounds.

3. Place the cookies into the pre-heated oven and bake for around 10 minutes. The cookies will go a lovely golden brown and will still be soft to the touch but will firm up as they cool on a wire rack. The outside of the cookies should be crunchy with a lovely chewy centre.

4. My favourite and very simple addition is to throw in a handful of dark chocolate bits to the mixture when I add the cornflakes, but be as adventurous as you like. I have to say that I do seem to keep returning to the original recipe which is so truly simple and also excessively moreish.

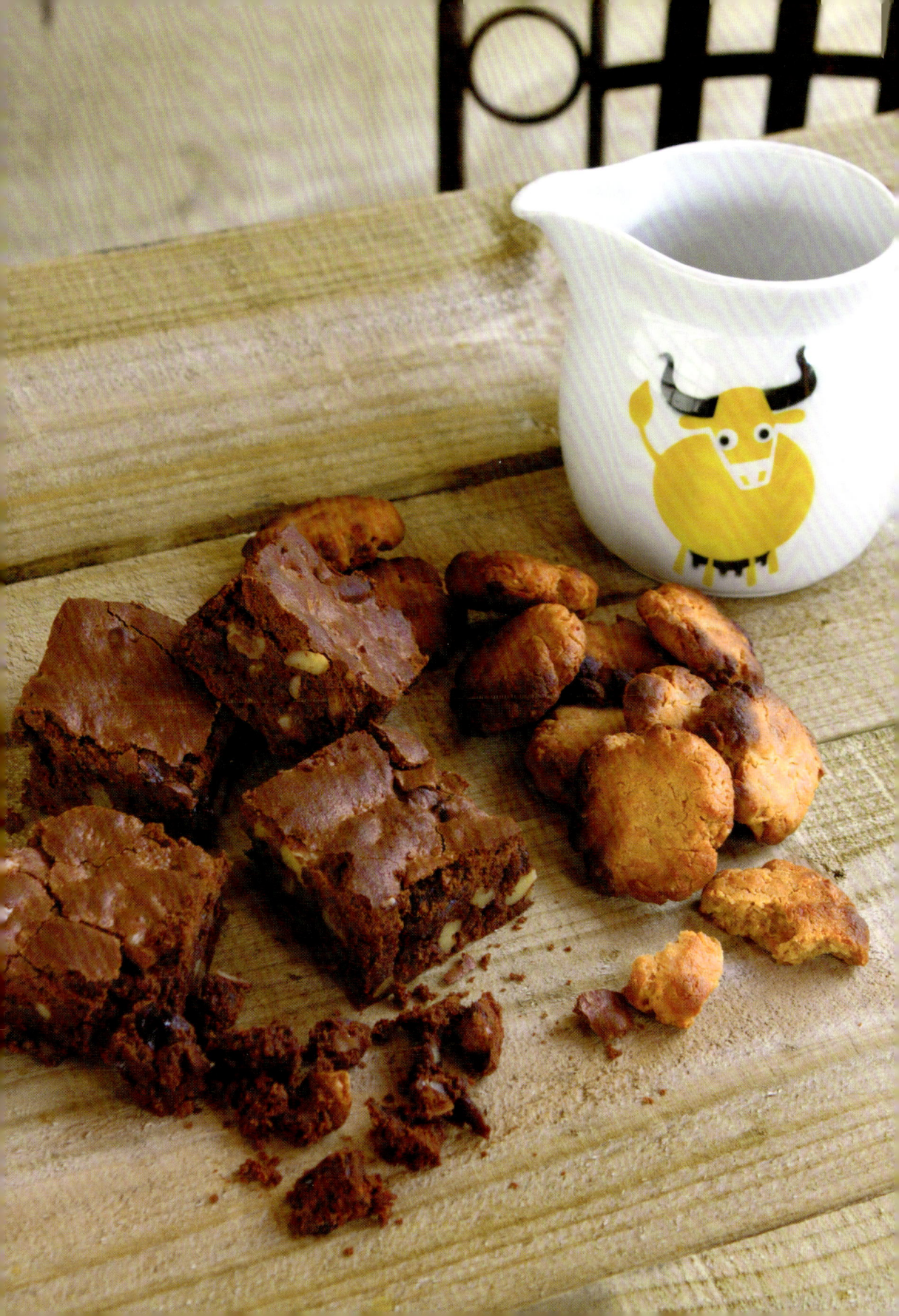

Banana and pecan cupcakes

— MAKES 18 —

I like to bake my cupcakes in the gorgeous rigid paper cases that are now so readily available. They are taller than a traditional patty-pan case, and help make the final result look much more professional.

CUPCAKES

125 grams (½ cup) of softened unsalted butter

160 grams (¾ cup) of golden caster sugar

5 grams (1 teaspoon) of vanilla bean paste

1 egg

2 very ripe bananas

135 grams (1 cup) of super-fine white rice flour

65 grams (½ cup) of glutinous rice flour

15 grams (3 teaspoons) of gluten free baking powder

¼ teaspoon of bicarbonate of soda

63mL (¼ cup) of milk

130 grams (4.6 ounces) of roughly chopped pecans

CARAMEL PECANS

18 pecan halves

4 tablespoons of golden caster sugar

CREAM CHEESE ICING

180 grams (6.3 ounces) of softened cream cheese

230 grams (1½ cups) of icing sugar

5 grams (1 teaspoon) of vanilla bean paste

Zest of a lemon, finely grated

1. Place a shelf in the middle of your oven before preheating to a temperature of 170°C/340°F. If you are using the rigid paper cases then simply place twenty of these evenly spaced on a baking tray and set aside while you prepare your mixture. If you are using the less rigid cases I'd suggest you place them into a muffin tin to give them some extra support during the filling and cooking process.

2. Place the softened butter, sugar and vanilla bean paste into the bowl of your bench-top mixer. With the whisk attachment secured, start at a low speed to roughly incorporate the ingredients before turning to the highest speed setting and allowing it to beat until the mixture is white and fluffy. You may need to stop the mixer occasionally to scrape down the sides.

3. If you don't have a bench-top mixer then you can cream these ingredients by hand with a wooden spoon or with a pair of hand-held rotary beaters.

4. You can check if the mixture is ready by rubbing a small amount between your thumb and forefinger – you shouldn't be able to feel the sugar crystals anymore as they will have dissolved.

5. Once the mixture is ready, add in the egg and again beat on the highest speed setting until completely incorporated and the mixture has returned to its fluffy texture.

6. Place the flesh from your two bananas into a small bowl and mash them with a fork until smooth. Now, remove the bowl with the egg and butter mixture from your mixer and add the mashed banana. With a wooden spoon, mix until the banana is completely incorporated.

7. Place a sieve over the mixing bowl and sift in the rice flours and baking powder.

8. Measure the milk into a small bowl and sprinkle over the bicarbonate of soda. Give this a quick stir before adding it to the other ingredients.

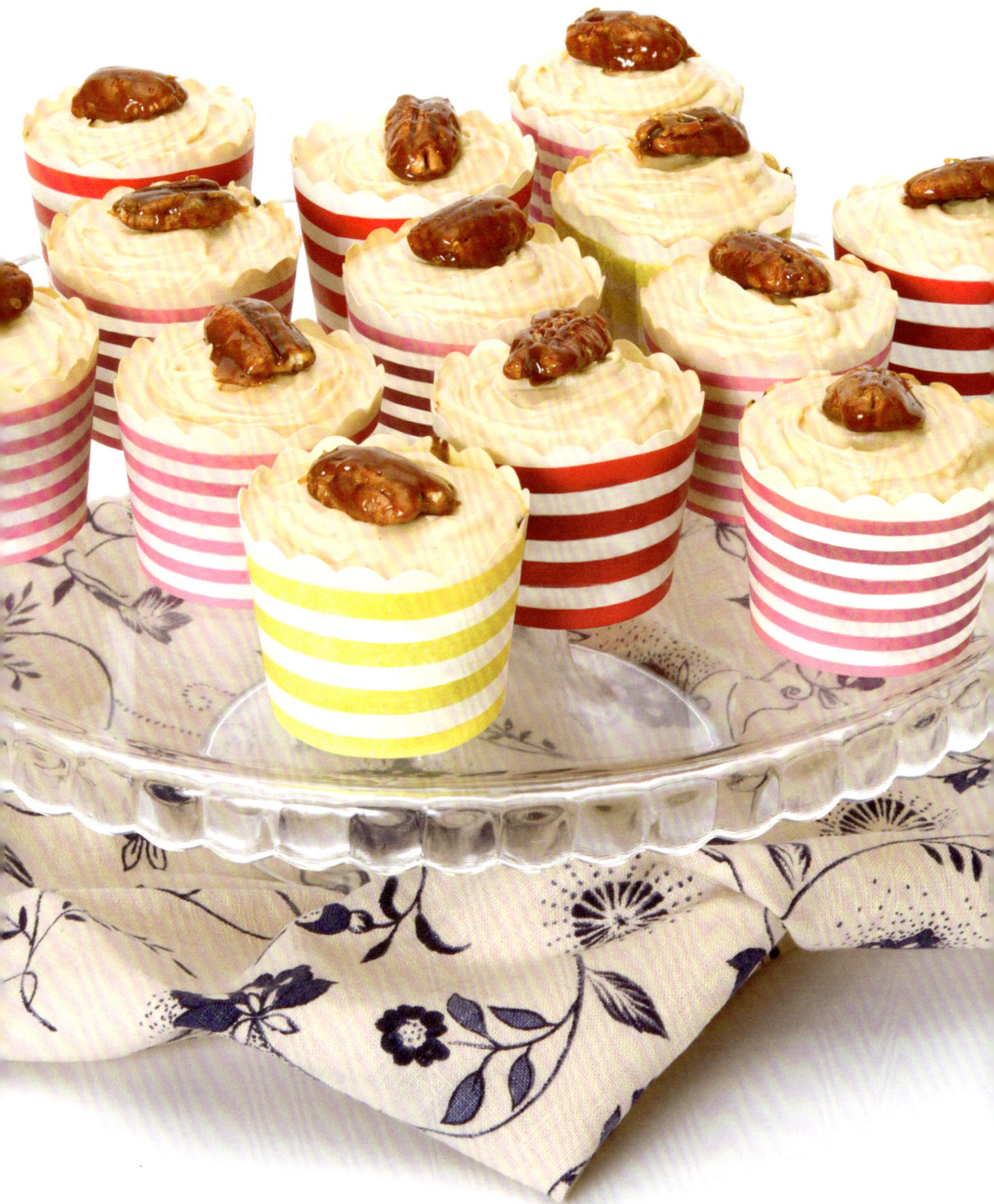

9. Mix the batter with the wooden spoon until all the ingredients are combined and the mixture is a smooth and consistent texture. Now add the pecans and stir them through the mixture so they are evenly distributed.

10. Use two teaspoons — one to scoop up the mixture and the other to scrape the mixture off the first spoon — and let the batter fall into the bottom of each cupcake case. I usually put a heaped teaspoon in each case then come back and add another. Then I have a look at all of the cases and add or remove mixture until they all contain the same amount — they'll be about ¾ full. Be sure to use the teaspoons to jiggle the mixture down into the bottom of the cases so that you don't leave any large air pockets which will cause your cupcakes to rise unevenly.

11. Place the cupcakes into the preheated oven for around 12 minutes until golden brown on top. You can check if they are cooked by placing a wooden skewer into the centre of a couple of cakes. If it comes out clean then they are ready. Once cooked, remove the tray from the oven, place the cupcakes onto a wire rack and leave them to cool.

12. Place a square of baking paper on a plate ready for the caramelised pecans. Place the golden caster sugar into a small non-stick saucepan and place it on a medium heat. Every so often give the pan a shake to keep the sugar from caramelizing unevenly — you will first start to see the sugar turning to a liquid around the edges of the pan so take a spoon and just move the sugar around to allow it to continue to melt evenly. Don't stir the sugar as it may crystallise but rather imagine you're making an omelette and you just want to agitate the sugar as it colours.

13. Once the sugar is completely melted, keep it on the heat until you have achieved a rich golden colour — similar to the colour of golden syrup. If you get much darker than this the caramel will taste burnt rather than having that slight bitter edge everyone loves so much.

14. As soon as the caramel is ready, remove the pan from the heat and add the pecan halves. With a fork, toss the pecans in the caramel to coat them and as each one is coated remove it and place it flat side down on the waiting baking paper. You'll need to move fairly quickly here as the caramel will start to set quickly. Once all the pecans are covered in their golden coating set them aside to cool and set into crunchy morsels.

15. Once the cupcakes have cooled completely you can prepare the icing. Into a medium bowl place the softened cream cheese, vanilla bean paste and lemon zest. Beat these with a handheld rotary beater until they are light before gradually adding the icing sugar until completely combined. The mixture will be light and creamy with a hint of zing from the lemon zest.

16. Ice each cupcake and adorn with a caramel pecan in the centre of each. If you serve these immediately, the caramel will be crunchy and provide a lovely textural contrast to the soft moist cake. However, I often prepare these in advance and simply place them in an airtight container until required. In this instance, the moisture from the icing will melt the caramel and create a beautiful swirl over the top of the cake with the pecan remaining the focal point in the centre. Either way is delicious, and both look just as appealing, so it really depends on how you prefer to serve them.

Marmalade and polenta cookies

— MAKES 36 —

These little biscuits look a little like those jam drops of old but the crunch that the polenta brings, along with the lovely slightly bitter flavour of the marmalade, makes for quite an adult little biscuit. I usually make these with my homemade very fine-cut blood orange marmalade, which not only tastes beautiful, but has the added benefit of a rich amber colour.

170 grams (⅔ cup) of unsalted butter, softened

170 grams (¾ cup) of golden caster sugar

255 grams (1⅓ cup) of fine grain polenta (corn meal)

100 grams (¾ cup) of super-fine white rice flour

Finely grated zest of 3 oranges

2 eggs, lightly whisked

A jar of good quality orange marmalade

1. Grease and line three baking sheets and set them aside while you prepare the biscuit mixture.

2. Place all the ingredients, except for the marmalade, into a large mixing bowl and stir thoroughly to combine into a soft, grainy, orange-scented mixture.

3. Take teaspoon sized amounts of the mixture and roll it between your palms to create balls that are about 1½cm (1 inch) in diameter. Place them on the lined baking trays leaving adequate spacing (about 4 cm or 1½ inches apart) as they will spread when they are baked.

4. Once you have rolled all the balls, gently push down on the centre of each to create a thumb-sized indentation in the top. Fill each of these indentations with some of the orange marmalade, trying to keep to the centre of the rounds.

5. Place the trays into the refrigerator for at least one hour so the mixture can chill before baking. This will reduce the amount of spread when the trays are placed in the oven.

6. After the biscuits have been in the refrigerator for 30 minutes place a shelf in the middle of your oven and preheat to a temperature of 180°C/355°F.

7. Place the trays in the preheated oven and bake for around 6 minutes until the edges are lightly golden. Remove the biscuits and leave them to cool for around 5 minutes on the tray before moving them to a wire rack to finish cooling to room temperature.

Pikelets

I still think the classics are often the best so I like to serve my pikelets with slightly salted butter and some good homemade apricot jam.

95 grams (⅔ cup) of super-fine white rice flour

45 grams (⅓ cup) of glutinous rice flour

A pinch of salt

40 grams (2 tablespoons) of golden caster sugar

10 grams (2 teaspoons) of gluten free baking powder

¼ teaspoon of bicarbonate of soda

1 egg

250mL (1 cup) of milk

Juice of ½ a lemon

40 grams (2 tablespoons) of melted butter

Extra butter, for frying

1. Add the lemon juice to the milk and stir to combine before setting it aside until required.

2. Add the flours, sugar, baking powder and bicarb into a large mixing bowl and stir with a wooden spoon to ensure they are well combined. Make a well in the centre of the bowl ready for the wet mixture.

3. Take the milk that you had placed aside and add the egg and melted butter. With a fork, whisk them to combine well and then pour the mixture into the centre of the dry ingredients. Using the wooden spoon, gradually combine the ingredients. To minimise the risk of a lumpy batter use the spoon to gradually draw in the flour from the edge of the well as you stir. If you end up with a few lumps, don't worry you can easily squash them on the side of the bowl.

4. Heat a heavy-based frying pan over a medium heat. Once hot, add a little of the extra butter to the pan and move it around to coat the surface. Add tablespoonfuls of mixture to the pan – I usually do three in a batch and cook until bubbly on top and golden brown underneath. Flip the pikelets over and cook briefly on the other side until lightly golden. Transfer the pikelets to a clean tea (dish) towel and lightly wrap them up while you continue cooking the remaining batches. Keep the pikelets wrapped in the towel to make sure they are nice and moist until required.

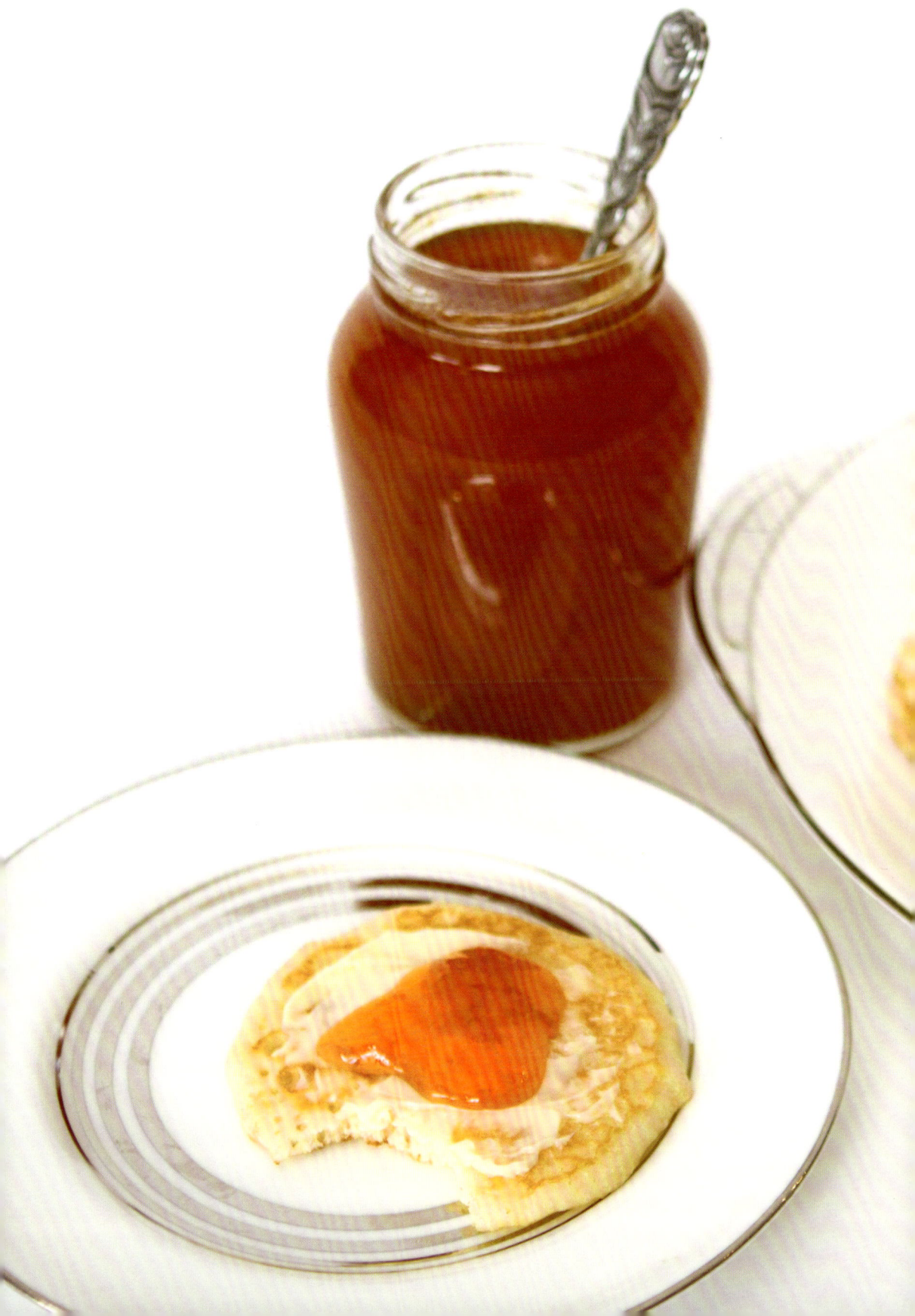

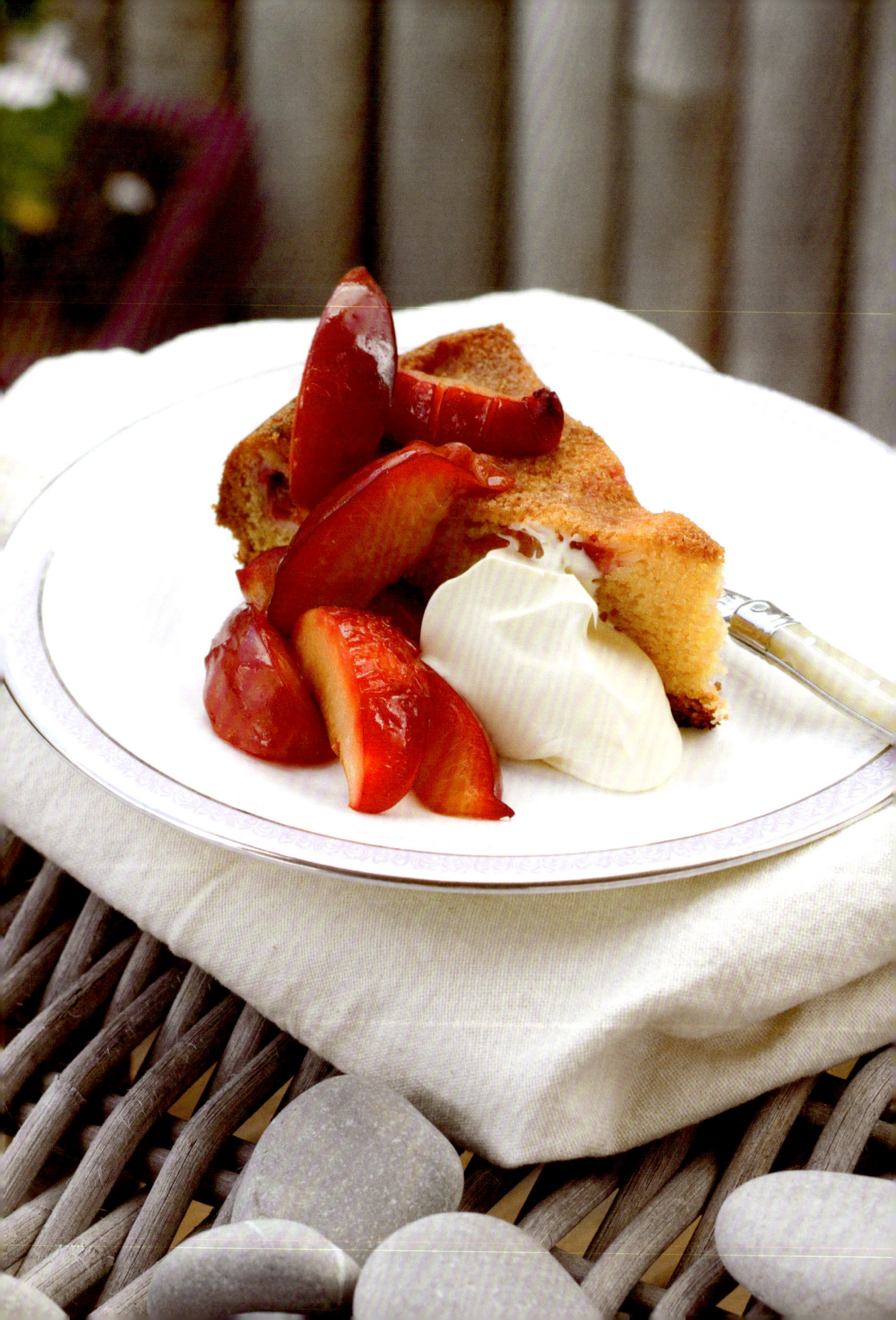

Fresh summer plum cake

— SERVES 12 —

I love the look of a slice of this cake on a plain white plate. The plums tend to sink through the cake batter as it cooks and the pigment in the skins turn a beautiful vibrant pink that contrasts perfectly with the pale yellow of the cake. The smell of the cooked fruit almost makes me heady as I think of long summer days lounging in the sunshine eating fresh plums and licking my fingers clean of all the sticky goodness.

500 grams (1.5 pounds) of ripe summer plums, halved and stoned

150 grams (⅔ cup) of softened unsalted butter

160 grams (¾ cup) of golden caster sugar

5 grams (1 teaspoon) of vanilla bean paste

3 eggs

145 grams (1 cup) of super-fine white rice flour

75 grams (½ cup) of glutinous rice flour

20 grams (4 teaspoons) of gluten free baking powder

100mL (5 tablespoons) of milk

1. Place a shelf in the middle of your oven before preheating to a temperature of 170°C/340°F. Grease a 23cm (9 inch) spring-form cake tin with butter and then line the base with grease-proof paper.

2. Place the softened butter, sugar and vanilla bean paste into the bowl of your bench-top mixer. With the whisk attachment secured, start at a low speed to roughly incorporate the ingredients before turning to the highest speed setting and allowing it to beat until the mixture is white and fluffy. You may need to stop the mixer occasionally to scrape down the sides.

3. If you don't have a bench-top mixer then you can cream these ingredients by hand with a wooden spoon or with a pair of hand-held rotary beaters.

4. You can check if the mixture is ready by rubbing a small amount between your thumb and forefinger — you shouldn't be able to feel the sugar crystals anymore as they will have dissolved.

5. Once the mixture is ready, add the eggs one at a time, beating until each is completely incorporated and the mixture has returned to its fluffy texture.

6. Place a sieve over the mixing bowl and sift in the rice flours and baking powder. Add the milk and mix the batter with a wooden spoon until all the ingredients are combined and the mixture is a smooth and consistent texture.

7. Spoon two-thirds of the cake batter into the bottom of the tin and spread it out so that it evenly covers the base. Arrange the plum halves on top of the cake batter in one even layer and then spread the remaining batter in a thin layer over the fruit.

8. Place the cake in the pre-heated oven and bake for around 40 minutes. You can check if the cake is cooked by placing a wooden skewer into the centre and if it comes out clean then it is ready. It will also have just started to pull away from the sides of the tin. Leave the cake to cool for around 15 minutes before removing the collar from the tin.

9. This cake may be served warm or at room temperature but always with a good dollop of beautifully luscious clotted cream.

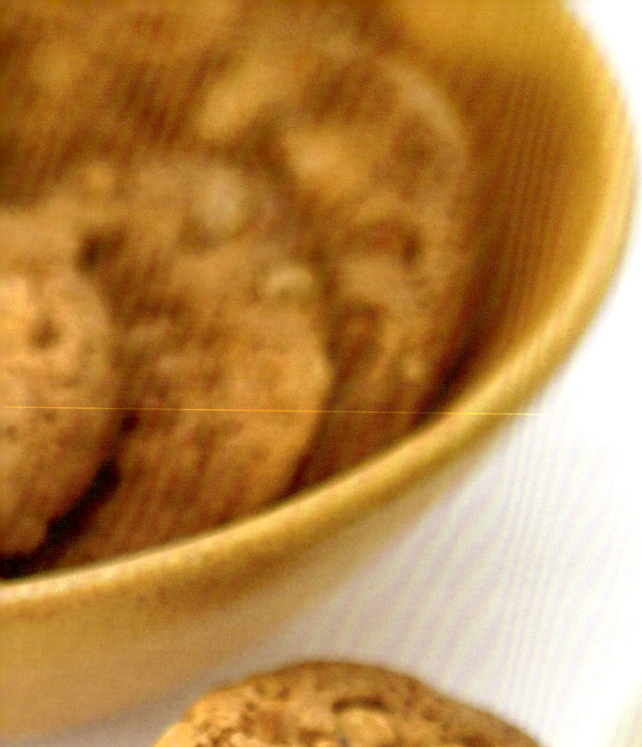

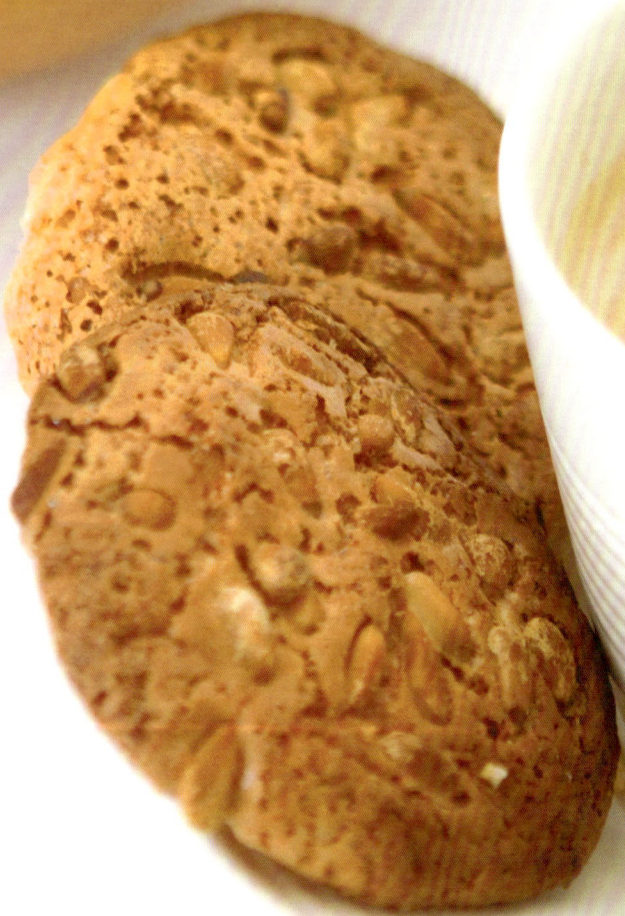

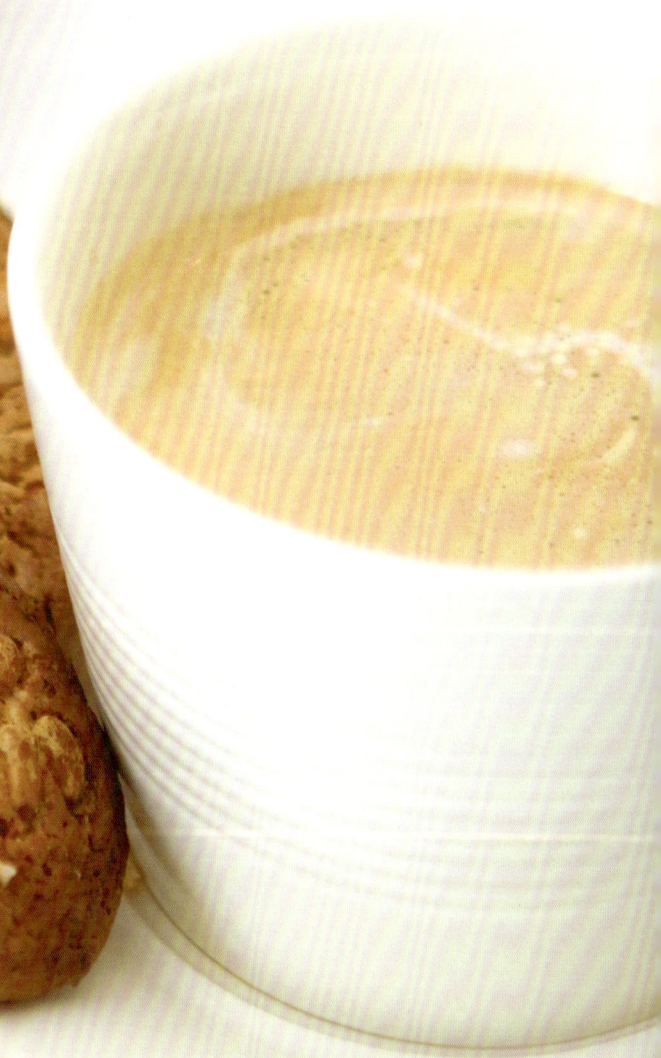

Corsican macarons

— MAKES 12 —

I was watching a documentary one day about Corsica and the presenter was talking about the main crops that are grown on that island. He was walking through a beautiful forest of chestnut trees picking the shiny brown-shelled nuts out of their spiky casing while talking about the sweet flour that is made, as well as the other main crops of pine-nuts and citrus fruits. It reminded me that I had some chestnut flour in the pantry and he inspired me to see what I could come up with. This recipe is the result of that exploration.

200 grams (1 cup) of golden caster sugar

100 grams (1 cup) of chestnut flour

20 grams (1 tablespoon) of super-fine white rice flour

Finely grated zest of 1 orange

2 egg whites

50 grams of pine-nuts

1. Place a shelf in the middle of your oven before preheating to a temperature of 170°C/340°F. Grease and line a baking sheet and set it aside while you prepare the macaron mixture.

2. Into a large mixing bowl place the flours, sugar and orange zest. Give the dry ingredients a good mix so the orange zest is well distributed.

3. Place the egg whites in a medium mixing bowl and, using a hand-held electric or rotary beater, whip them until they are frothy and almost reaching the soft peak stage.

4. Using a large metal spoon, take half the egg whites and fold them through the chestnut flour mixture until well combined. Add the remaining egg white and fold through the mixture until well combined and smooth.

5. Drop the mixture onto the lined baking tray in about 2 teaspoonful rounds. The mixture will spread considerably during baking so leave a large amount of space between the macarons. Sprinkle the pine-nuts on top of the macaron rounds before placing them in the oven to bake for around 20 minutes until golden brown.

6. Remove the tray from the oven and leave the macarons to sit for a couple of minutes so they start to cool and firm up a little. Very gently remove the macarons from the tray and leave them to cool on a wire rack. These rather adult biscuits are a lovely accompaniment to a good strong espresso.

Lunches

IN OUR WORLD of busy hither and thither, I feel that in some ways lunch has become the lost meal. Many of us work in offices or factories located in large multi-storey buildings where it is so easy to lose track of the natural flow of each day.

On the weekend though, my husband and I always try to make sure we sit down together for every meal and our lunches are usually delicious and greatly anticipated. Often we're out and about running errands or catching up with friends having lunch in a cafe, but for me the best lunches are those we make together at home.

On a Saturday morning we usually do our grocery shopping. Our local farmer's market is held on the third Saturday of the month. These Saturday's are blissfully relaxed and filled with simple indulgence. We come home, our bags laden with the most beautiful produce anyone could ever wish for and our two dogs bounce around as we carry our treasure into the house. The stereo goes on and we unpack our winnings while discussing the beautiful meals we'll be preparing over the coming week.

Then, while my husband gives the dogs some much needed (and deserved) attention I start to prepare our lunch. Maybe some of those incredible heritage tomatoes we bought from Robbie, the purple basil that has just started flowering and that ball of buffalo mozzarella we just had to buy. I start to slice the tomatoes — green zebra, college challenger, hillbilly and grosse lisse varieties. By now the dog's need for attention has been assuaged and my husband comes to join me — he starts to pick off the basil leaves and scatter them roughly torn over the multi-coloured slices of tomato. I tear the buffalo mozzarella apart and gently lay pieces of the pure white creamy yet slightly rubbery cheese around the platter. Plenty of salt and pepper followed by a generous drizzle of balsamic and then some herby green olive oil, a final flourish of basil flowers and a basket of bread and our meal is ready.

The simplicity of these moments is what I crave, the enjoyment of a beautiful summer day in the best way possible: love — of people, of food, of producers and of course, of our darling doggies!

Corn and avocado salsa

— SERVES 6 —

The sweet burst of flavour as the corn kernels pop in my mouth always make me smile when I eat this salsa and the refreshing nature of cucumber makes for a wonderful combination. I seem to always feel lighter and fresher after I eat this salsa — I think it is just the simplicity of the ingredients and the way they all work together that makes this such a pleasure to eat.

1 Spanish (red) onion, finely chopped

20 grams (1 tablespoon) of golden caster sugar

80mL (4 tablespoons) of red wine vinegar

3 large corn cobs with husks still intact

2 large ripe avocados

2 Lebanese (or small) cucumbers

4 tomatoes

A handful of chopped mint

A handful of chopped coriander

Extra virgin olive oil

Salt and pepper

1. Place the finely chopped onion, sugar and vinegar into a large mixing bowl. Give these a good stir so the onion pieces separate and the vinegar and sugar are evenly distributed. Set the bowl aside while you prepare the other ingredients. This will give the onion time to soak up the sugar and vinegar which will allow it to soften and cut through the astringency that raw onion can sometimes bring to a dish.

2. Place your corn cobs onto the turntable of your microwave and cook them on high for 9 minutes. If you can't fit them all in together then just cook each one separately for 3 minutes. Once the corn cobs are cooked, remove them from the microwave and set them aside to cool down a little before handling.

3. While the corn cobs are cooling, dice the avocados, tomatoes and cucumber into 1.5 - 2cm (½ inch) pieces. Add the vegetables to the mixing bowl with the onion and vinegar and stir gently to combine while trying to keep the pieces of avocado intact.

4. When the corn cobs are cool enough to handle, pull the husks from the corn cobs and remove as much of the silk as possible. To remove the kernels from the corn cob, stand it on its end on your chopping board then with a sharp knife cut downwards between the core and the kernels. Repeat this process all the way around each of the cobs and add the kernels to the other ingredients in the bowl.

5. Combine the coriander and mint with the other ingredients along with enough olive oil to make the salsa glisten. Season with salt and pepper before serving.

Green bean, artichoke and avocado salad

— SERVES 4 —

The onset of summer brings with it many culinary joys. For me, one of its great veggie heroes is the humble and often overlooked green bean. This salad celebrates the crispy sweetness of these pods by combining them with the flavours of honey, toasted almonds and marinated Persian feta.

THE VINAIGRETTE:

190mL (¾ cup) of extra virgin olive oil

65mL (¼ cup) of white wine vinegar

20mL (1 tablespoon) of Dijon mustard

20mL (1 tablespoon) of honey

Salt and pepper

THE SALAD:

800 grams (1 pound 12 ounces) of green beans

8 roasted artichoke hearts

2 avocados

120 grams (4 ounces) of Persian feta

80 grams (3 ounces) of flaked almonds

Salt and pepper

Place all the ingredients in a clean and dry jar with a metal lid. Season with salt and pepper, remembering that it is always better to under season and then make adjustments. Put the lid back on the jar and shake it vigorously until all the ingredients are emulsified. Taste and then adjust the seasoning. The vinaigrette will keep in the jar at room temperature for a couple of weeks.

THE SALAD

1. Bring a saucepan of water to the boil and then season with salt — it should taste like the sea. Cut the tops off the beans and then place them in the rapidly boiling water. Place the lid back on the saucepan to bring it back to the boil as soon as possible. Let the beans cook for around 1 to 2 minutes — it depends how crunchy you want them, but no more than 2 minutes. Immediately drain them and plunge them into ice cold water to set the colour and stop them from cooking.

2. Place a small frying pan over a medium heat. Scatter the flaked almonds over the base of the pan and gently move them around with a wooden spoon. Once the almonds have turned a lovely pale golden colour remove the pan from the heat and immediately tip the nuts into a bowl to cool. Be sure to stay with the almonds while they are roasting as the natural oils will make them brown very quickly and if not watched will likely burn.

3. Cut the roasted artichoke hearts into sixths, peel the avocados and chop the flesh into 2cm (½ inch) chunks.

4. Place the beans, artichoke and avocado into a large mixing bowl. Shake up the vinaigrette in the jar and spoon 8 tablespoons over the ingredients. Season with salt and pepper and then gently toss the ingredients with your hands to ensure everything is coated in the beautiful vinaigrette. Be sure to taste and adjust the seasoning as required.

5. Place the salad in the centre of the serving plate, ensuring you achieve some height. Drizzle the salad with a little extra vinaigrette before crumbling the feta over the top and then finishing with a scattering of flaked almonds.

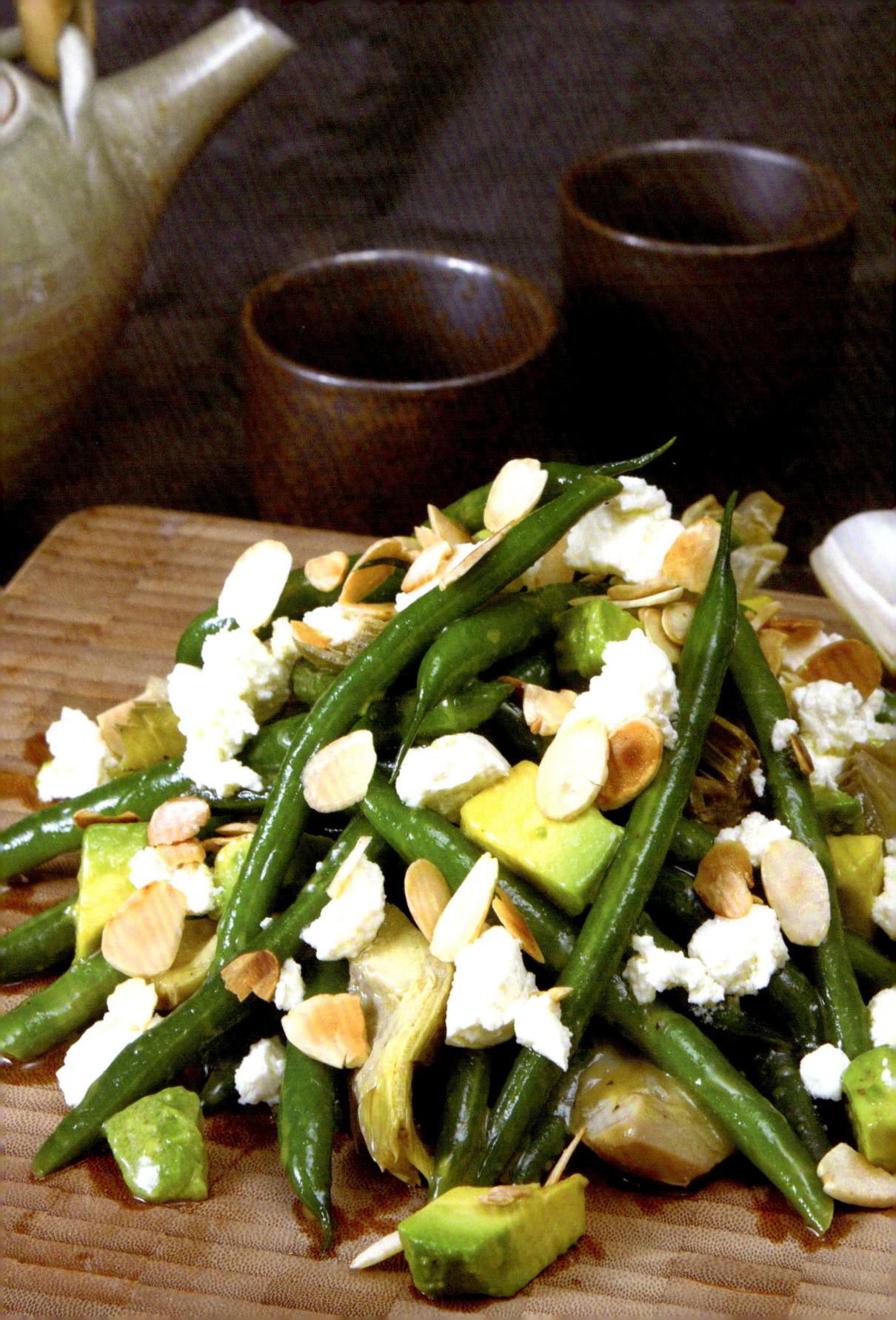

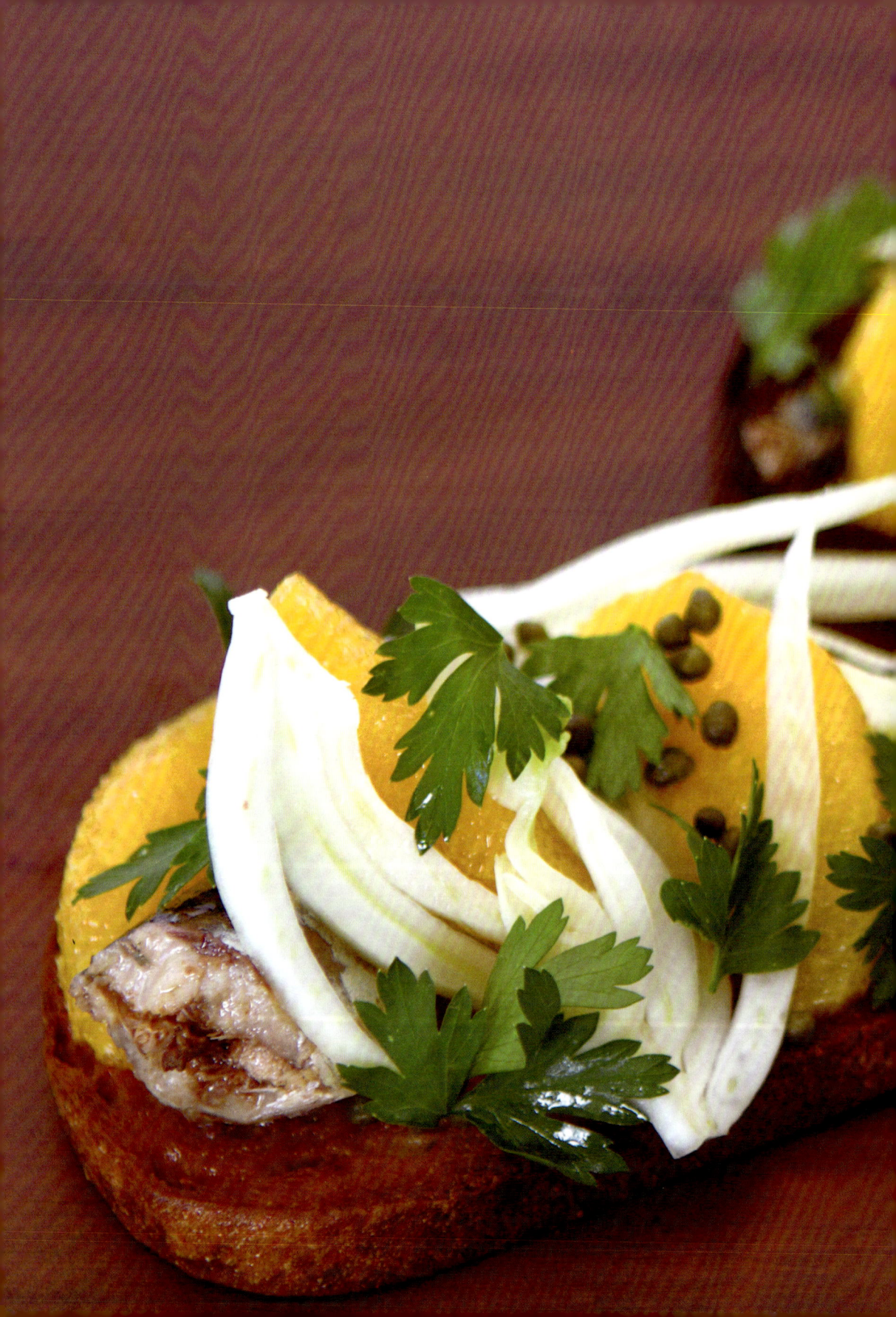

Bruschetta of sardines, oranges and fennel

— SERVES 4 —

Sardines often get a bad rap for being overly 'fishy' both in flavour and smell. If you're lucky enough to find some fresh sardines at your fishmonger then buy them immediately and simply rub them with thyme and lemon, season well and briefly cook them on the barbeque before digging in with your fingers. I like to use blood oranges when they are in season for their rich colour, but also because their sweet but slightly pithy flavour combines beautifully with the oily fish.

4 slices of good quality gluten free bread

4 x 90 gram (3 ounces) tins of good quality sardines in olive oil

4 small oranges

2 small fennel bulbs

4 tablespoons lilliput (extra fine) capers

A large handful of continental (flat leaf) parsley leaves

Extra virgin olive oil

Salt and pepper

1. Remove the core from the base of the fennel bulb and discard before finely slicing the fennel and placing it in a medium mixing bowl. Into the bowl add the capers, parsley leaves and the entire contents of the sardine tins (including the olive oil).

2. Take the orange and slice off the top and bottom of the skin so you can just see the flesh. Place the orange on one flat end and following the curve of the fruit with long slow movements from top to bottom remove all the skin and pith until you have a lovely ball of orange flesh.

3. With a small sharp knife, segment the orange into the mixing bowl with the other ingredients. To do this, cup the orange in the palm of your non-preferred hand and with the knife, cut down next to one of the ribs that run between each segment until you reach the heart of the orange. Repeat this on the other side of the rib and continue this right around the orange. This will provide you with beautiful crescents of juicy flesh without the tough membrane.

4. Once you have finished cutting out all the segments squeeze the juice out of the remaining membrane into the bowl over the other ingredients. Be sure to extract as much juice as possible before discarding.

5. In a medium frying pan add around 2 tablespoons of extra virgin olive oil and place on a medium heat. Once heated, place the slices of bread in the centre of the pan and leave them to turn a beautiful golden brown before turning and allowing the other side to also brown. Remove the bread from the pan and place in the centre of the serving plate.

6. Return to the bowl containing all the other ingredients and season them with salt and pepper before gently tossing them with your hands to ensure everything is coated in the lovely orange olive oil. Taste and adjust the seasoning before mounding the salad on top of the waiting bread – you should have plenty of height. Scatter with a couple of extra parsley leaves and serve.

Poached chicken with mango mayonnaise

This is one of those recipes that I return to time and time again. Its simplicity belies the elegance and sophistication of the final dish. Each summer we go to an evening production of Shakespeare in the Melbourne Royal Botanical Gardens – my favourite of his plays: A Midsummer Night's Dream. This dish is a regular at these gatherings and one that always generates the requisite praise.

THE CHICKEN

2 kilogram (4 pound) roasting chicken

1 onion, studded with 2 whole cloves

2 carrots cut into quarters

1 celery stick cut into pieces

2 garlic cloves

A bouquet garni (a sprig of thyme, a bay leaf and several sprigs of parsley)

3 sprigs of fresh tarragon

375mL (1½ cups) of dry white wine

Salt

6 whole black peppercorns

1. Wash the chicken inside and out in cold running water and then place it, breast side down, in a pot just large enough to hold it.

2. Add the onion, carrots, celery, garlic, bouquet garni, tarragon, peppercorns and salt to the pot. Pour in the wine and enough water so that about three quarters of the chicken is immersed. The breast meat should be completely submerged.

3. Bring the covered pot just to the boil and then simmer gently for 45 minutes before carefully turning the bird over so the breast is now on top. Continue to gently simmer for around another 45 minutes until the chicken is tender. To check that the meat is cooked through pierce the thigh with a skewer and ensure the juice runs clear not pink.

4. Turn off the heat and leave the chicken to cool in the stock. Remove the chicken from the broth once it has cooled to room temperature. Strain the stock through a fine sieve and utilise for other recipes. I usually measure amounts of 500mL (2 cups) into plastic containers and place them in the freezer. Remove the skin from the chicken, cut into portions and place them on your serving platter.

THE MAYONNAISE

2 egg yolks, at room temperature

5mL (1 teaspoon) of tarragon infused Dijon mustard

Salt and pepper

250mL (1 cup) of peanut oil

40mL (2 tablespoons) of white wine vinegar

1 large ripe mango

½ teaspoon of cayenne pepper

1 tablespoon of finely chopped tarragon

1. Place the egg yolks, mustard and a little salt and pepper into a mixing bowl. Place a tea (dish) towel on your bench to prevent the bowl from sliding. Use a balloon whisk to mix the ingredients in the bowl until they are well combined.

2. Now start to add the oil in a thin trickle while continuing to whisk. As the mayonnaise begins to thicken, add the oil in a steady stream while continuing to whisk all the time. When you have incorporated all the oil, whisk vigorously for 30 seconds until the mayonnaise is thick and glossy. Add the vinegar and then taste for seasoning.

3. Remove the skin from the mango and cut the flesh from the stone. Place the mango flesh, cayenne pepper, tarragon and mayonnaise into a food processor and pulse until smooth. Drizzle half the mayonnaise over the prepared chicken and place the remainder in a small bowl to serve.

4. If mangoes are out of season you can use a tin of drained mango cheeks although the flavour will not be as intense and fresh. I often purchase a box of perfectly ripe mangoes during Summer and after removing the skin I cut the flesh away from the stone. I then place the flesh from each mango into a snap lock freezer bag and place in the freezer ready for use during the cooler months.

> If you don't have any tarragon mustard then plain Dijon is a good alternative. Just add some extra fresh tarragon to your mayonnaise to enhance the flavour.

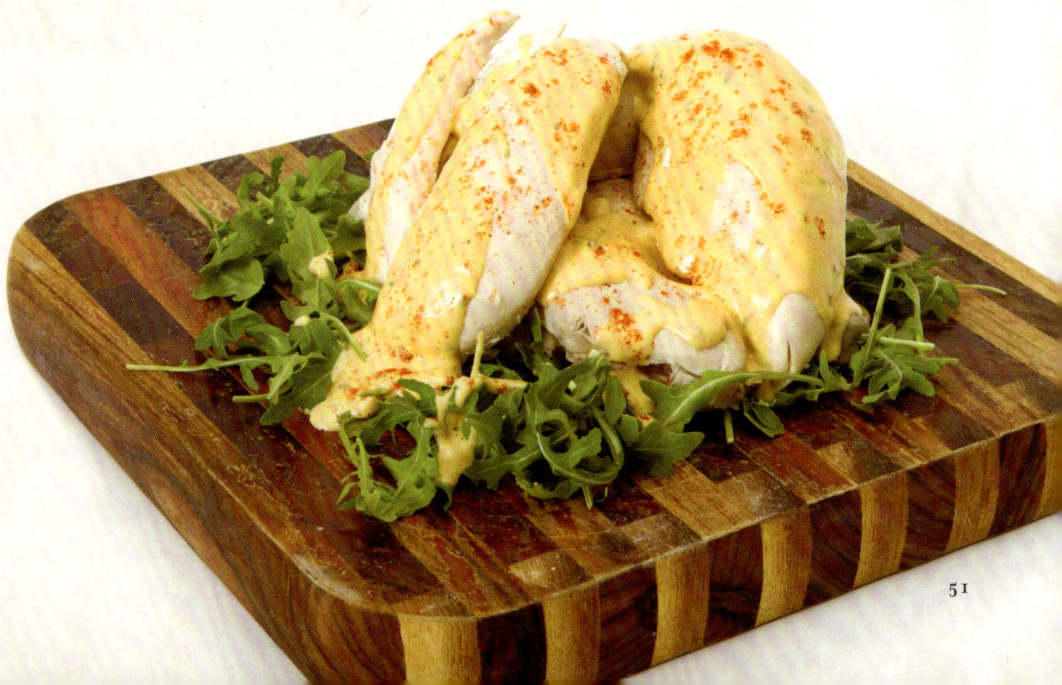

Potato salad

— SERVES 6 —

Some people like an oil based potato salad but I cannot resist a beautiful mayonnaise and sour cream dressing. The creaminess of this salad is cut by the subtle onion flavour of the chives and the addition of perfectly cooked hardboiled eggs not only looks beautiful when sliced and laid over the top of the salad, but the slightly grainy and velvety texture of the egg yolk is a wonderful accompaniment to the waxy potatoes.

20 kipfler potatoes or any other waxy variety

6 eggs

Half a bunch of fresh chives

Half a bunch of fresh parsley, finely chopped

125 grams (½ cup) of sour cream

125 grams (½ cup) of mayonnaise

Salt and pepper

1. Boil the potatoes whole in their skins until cooked.

2. Remove the potatoes from the water and add the eggs. Cook the eggs in boiling water for 10-12 minutes.

3. Dice the potatoes into good sized pieces while the eggs are cooking.

4. While the potatoes are still warm add the remaining ingredients (except the eggs) and stir gently to combine. I just snip the chives in with my kitchen scissors.

5. Season to taste and then spoon into your serving dish. Slice the eggs into quarters and arrange on top of the potatoes.

6. Chill until ready to serve.

Caprese salad

There is almost nothing more appetising to me than a bowl of pristine heirloom tomatoes picked at their perfect level of ripeness under the hot Australian Summer sun. The heady smell of their leaves and the furry texture of their stems coupled with the smooth firmness of the fruit makes me smile every time. This is so simple I almost feel guilty for writing it down.

8 perfectly ripe summer tomatoes

125 grams (4.4 ounces) of buffalo mozzarella

A handful of basil leaves

Balsamic vinegar

Extra virgin olive oil

Salt and pepper

1. Cut your tomatoes into various shapes. Slice the large ones into thick slices and place them over the bottom of your serving plate. Cut the medium sized tomatoes into segments and the small cherry tomatoes can just be cut in half. Arrange these pieces over the top of the slices to amplify the natural beauty of these fruits. Season with salt and pepper before scattering the roughly torn basil leaves over the entire plate.

2. Take your beautiful soft ball of mozzarella and gently ease it apart with your fingers. Tear it into rustic bite sized pieces and lay these slightly oozing chunks over the tomatoes and basil leaves.

3. Drizzle over some balsamic vinegar and follow with a good lug of olive oil, being sure to lightly coat everything in the grassy golden liquid.

4. Serve immediately with some good quality bread to mop up the oily juices.

Nectarine, roquette and prosciutto salad with raspberry vinaigrette

— SERVES 4 —

The sweetness of raspberries coupled with the acidity of vinegar and the mild background heat of the Dijon mustard combine to create a lovely and sumptuous dressing for this elegant salad.

1 punnet of raspberries

40mL (2 tablespoons) of white wine vinegar

2.5mL (½ teaspoon) of Dijon mustard

80mL (4 tablespoons) of extra virgin olive oil

Salt and pepper

250 grams (9 ounces) of roquette (arugula)

4 white nectarines

8 thin slices of prosciutto

1 pomegranate

1. Tip the raspberries into a bowl and use a pestle or blunt kitchen instrument to grind them into a pulp. Place a fine sieve over a small mixing bowl and pour the raspberry pulp into the sieve. Work the berry pulp through the sieve so you end up with a smooth consistency. Add the mustard, vinegar and olive oil to the raspberry pulp and use a small balloon whisk to bring the dressing together. Season with salt and pepper and then set aside until later.

2. Arrange the roquette leaves on four individual plates to form a slightly mounded base for the other ingredients. Cut the nectarines into eighths and arrange them on each plate. Now take the prosciutto and cut each slice into three before draping the pieces around the plates, being sure to snuggle them in and around the nectarine slices.

3. Roll the pomegranate on your chopping board to help loosen the pulp shrouded seeds before cutting the fruit in half. I find the easiest way to remove the pomegranate seeds is to place the halved fruit over a bowl, cut side down, and use a wooden spoon to hit the back of the fruit and let the ruby jewels fall into the bowl.

4. Give the dressing a final whisk and check the seasoning before drizzling it over the salads. Scatter over the pomegranate seeds and serve immediately.

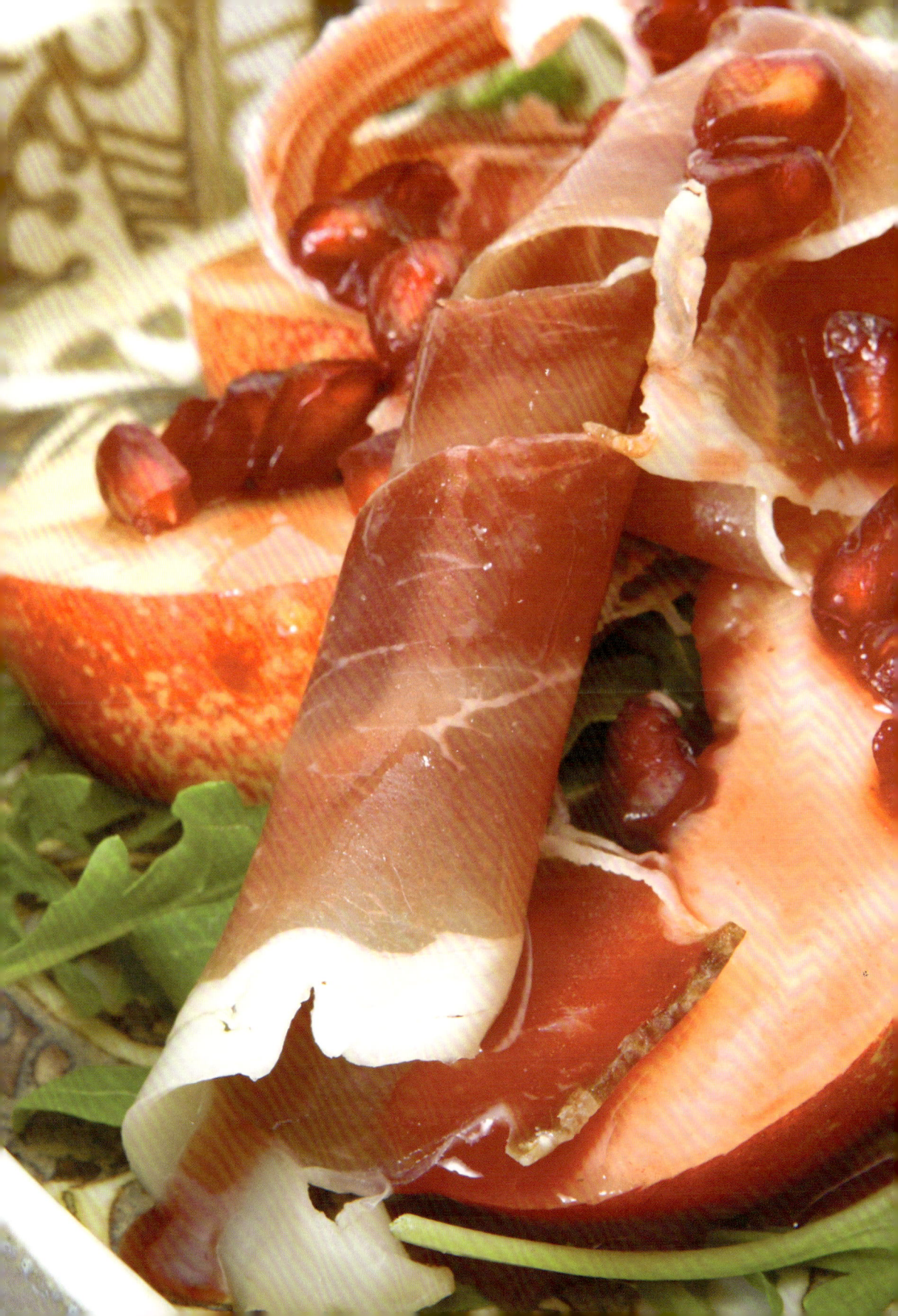

Apple, fennel, onion and roquette slaw

— SERVES 2 —

I have a wonderful handheld julienne slicer that I find perfect for cutting the apple into beautiful strips for this recipe. It looks just like a vegetable peeler but has teeth along the blade. Most kitchen stores will stock these and they do come in handy.

2 pink lady apples

1 baby fennel bulb

½ a Spanish (red) onion

50 grams (2 ounces) of roquette (arugula) leaves

30 grams (1 ounce) of walnuts, roughly chopped

60mL (3 tablespoons) of walnut oil

20mL (1 tablespoon) of white wine vinegar

20mL (1 tablespoon) of mayonnaise

Salt and pepper

1. Cut the apple into slices between 2 – 3mm (⅛ inch) in thickness. Then cut these into julienne (strips) of the same thickness. If you have a julienne slicer then this will make the job much quicker and easier but I still occasionally use a knife if I have time so I can practice my knife skills. Cut the fennel in a similar manner as well as the onion.

2. Add the julienned vegetables to a medium bowl along with the roquette leaves and give everything a gentle mix with your hands so the ingredients are evenly distributed. Add the walnuts, oil, vinegar, salt and pepper to the bowl and again mix gently to coat everything in the vinaigrette. Lastly add the mayonnaise and mix again before serving.

3. I enjoy eating this salad on its own but it also makes a wonderful accompaniment to some cold meats such as some rare roast beef accompanied by a little horseradish cream.

Savoury Things

WHEN I WAS about 14 years old and entering what I regard as one of the most challenging periods of my life, my teenage rebellion manifested in many ways. One of which was to disregard my gluten free diet.

I recall that during this period I truly believed I was invincible and my immune system appeared to cope extremely well with my daily gluten consumption - for a time at least. My desire to belong to the group, to be included and to be in no way special or different was strong — and what better way to achieve this than to eat whatever everyone else was eating.

I ate at fast food chains. I bought chocolate laden muffins from the school canteen. Pizza, hamburgers and fried chicken were all on the menu. It was wonderful.

At home I maintained the charade of a gluten free diet — the best of both worlds, tasty fast food with my friends and my mother's wonderful and creative cooking at home.

Eventually it all started to catch-up with me, I caught every cold, sore throat and stomach bug that passed through the school. I just didn't feel well. I was tired, irritable and I have no doubt that my poor diet contributed to my externally ebullient and internally depressive nature during this period of my life.

After a few years of gluten consumption, blood test results showed my mineral levels were rock-bottom. I was slowly but surely progressing down the path of malnutrition.

This is not an uncommon story, and I tell it not to shock but rather to highlight the importance food plays in our lives. It is not just a source of nutrients or something tasty to enjoy but it often binds people together. The ritual associated with sharing a meal along with the pleasure of a common experience all contribute to the fabric of our lives.

For someone who cannot eat gluten, the ability to share delicious food with others is just that bit harder, but with recipes that result in dishes of supreme quality they too can partake in these moments of communal pleasure.

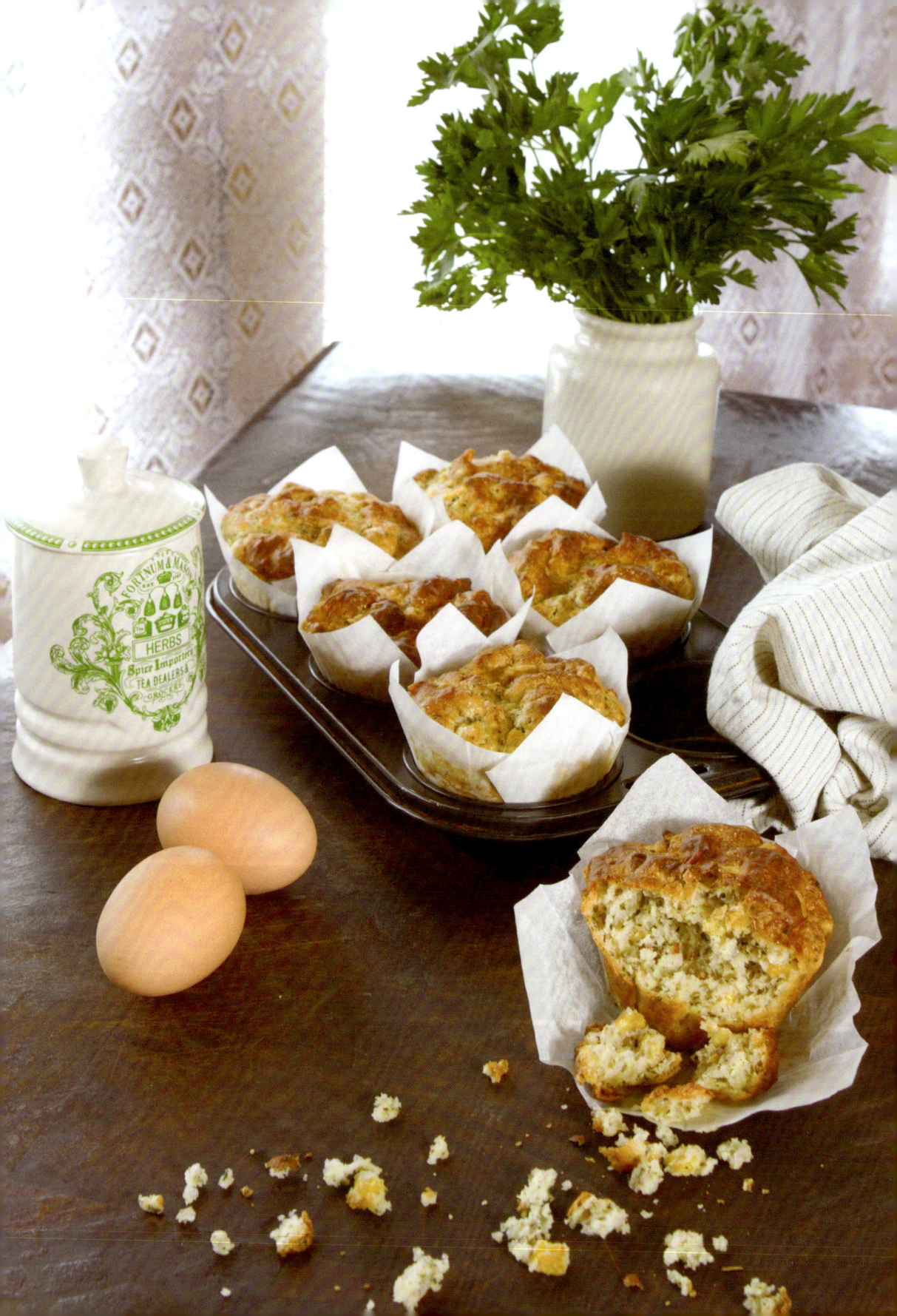

Cheesy corn and herb muffins

— MAKES 12 —

These muffins are best eaten while still slightly warm from the oven but they are also great to take to school or work as a mid-afternoon snack. I sometimes give them about 20 seconds in the microwave so I can enjoy that still warm experience.

200ml (¾ cup) of milk

Juice of half a lemon

150 grams (5 ounces) of corn kernels, fresh or frozen

150 grams (5 ounces) strong tasty cheese, grated

165 grams (1¼ cups) of super-fine white rice flour

85 grams (⅔ cup) of glutinous rice flour

20mL (4 teaspoons) of gluten free baking powder

2.5 grams (½ teaspoon) of bicarbonate of soda

1.25 grams (¼ teaspoon) of salt

20 grams (1 tablespoon) of dried oregano

10 grams (2 teaspoons) of dried rosemary

80 grams (⅓ cup) of unsalted butter, melted

2 eggs

1. Place a shelf in the middle of your oven before preheating to a temperature of 190°C/375°F. Line your muffin tin with 12 paper cases and set it aside until required.

2. If you are using frozen corn kernels remove them from the freezer and leave to defrost.

3. Pour the milk into a medium sized measuring jug (around 500mL or 2 cups capacity) and then add the lemon juice. Stir to combine and set the jug aside while you prepare the remaining ingredients.

4. Place the rice flours, baking powder, bicarbonate of soda, salt and herbs into a mixing bowl and stir them to combine. Add the corn kernels and cheese and mix them through the dry ingredients to ensure they are evenly distributed.

5. Crack the eggs into the milk and lemon juice mixture along with the melted butter and whisk everything together with a fork. Pour this mixture into the waiting ingredients in the mixing bowl. Mix all the ingredients together until well combined.

6. Using two spoons - one to scoop up the mixture and one to scrape the mixture off the first spoon, place a heaped tablespoon of mixture into each muffin case. If you have any mixture left over distribute it evenly between the muffin cases so they are all even in size.

7. Place the muffins into the preheated oven for around 18 minutes until golden brown on top. You can check if they are cooked by placing a wooden skewer into the centre of a couple of muffins. If it comes out clean then they are ready. Once cooked, remove the tray from the oven and let them cool for around 5 minutes in the tin before removing them to a wire rack to finish cooling.

Gougères

These golden puffs of cheesy goodness are the perfect accompaniment to a dry martini. The pâte à choux may be tightly covered and refrigerated for up to 12 hours before using, which makes these a perfect addition to any cocktail party menu.

250mL (1 cup) of water

¾ teaspoon of salt

110 grams (½ cup) of unsalted butter, cut into cubes

125 grams (1 cup) of super-fine white rice flour

5 eggs

110 grams (4 ounces) of gruyere cheese

1 egg, beaten and mixed with ½ teaspoon of salt for the glaze

40 - 60 grams (2 - 3 tablespoons) extra grated gruyere cheese

1. Place a shelf in the middle of your oven before preheating to a temperature of 200°C/390°F. Lightly butter a baking sheet and set it aside until required.

2. Place the water, salt and butter into a large saucepan and heat gently until the butter is melted. Bring it just up to the boil, then remove it from the heat and add the flour. Beat the mixture vigorously with a wooden spoon for a few moments until it pulls away from the sides of the saucepan and forms a ball. Keep beating the mixture for about a minute over a low heat to expel the excess moisture from the dough.

3. Crack one egg into a small bowl, give it a light whisk and set it aside until required. Crack an egg into the dough and beat it thoroughly until completely incorporated. Repeat this process with the remaining three eggs being sure to incorporate each into the dough before adding the next. Beat in enough of the reserved egg so the dough is shiny and just falls from the spoon. If too much egg is added, the dough will be too soft and won't hold its shape.

4. Rub the top of the dough with butter to prevent a skin from forming, and set it aside until cool.

Gougères are at their best served warm straight from the oven, but they can be baked ahead or stored in the freezer, and reheated in a low temperature oven.

5. Coarsely grate the Gruyère cheese and beat it into the cooled dough. Transfer the dough to a pastry bag fitted with a 1.25cm (½ inch) plain tip and pipe 4cm (1½ inch) mounds onto the baking sheet, spacing them well apart so they have space to puff during baking.

6. To make the glaze, crack the egg into a small bowl, add the salt and give it a good whisk to for the glaze. Brush the mounds with the egg glaze and sprinkle with the extra grated gruyère.

7. Bake for 25 to 30 minutes until the dough puffs and turns golden brown and crisp. The puffs often seem ready before time, so before you remove them from the oven take one out and let it cool for a minute or two to check if it is ready before removing the rest. It should stay crisp on the outside and slightly soft inside.

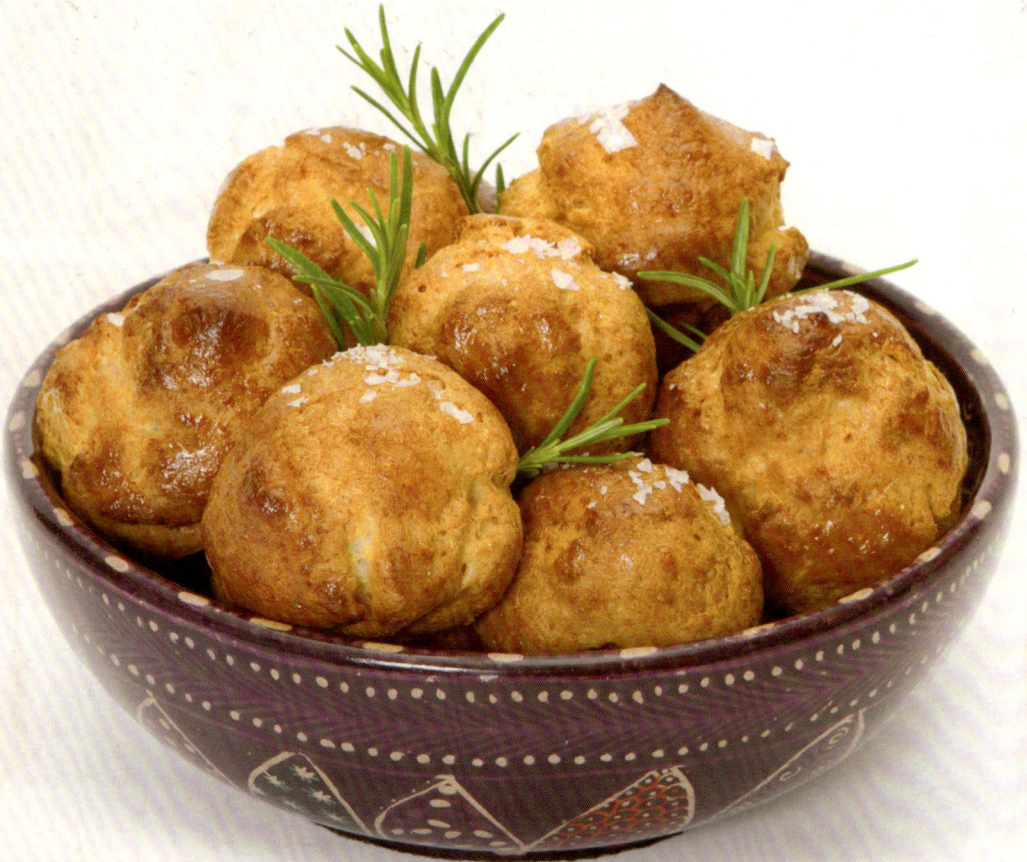

Pumpkin scones

Some people like to place a slice of cheese on freshly broken scones or sometimes a dollop of sour cream with a few chives. But for me the moist sweetness of these scones is beautifully accompanied by generous lashings of slightly salted butter and a pot of well brewed tea.

180 grams (1⅓ cups) of super-fine white rice flour

90 grams (⅔ cup) of glutinous rice flour

20 grams (4 teaspoons) of gluten free baking powder

½ teaspoon of cinnamon

¼ teaspoon of nutmeg

20 grams (1 tablespoon) of golden caster sugar

Pinch of salt

60 grams (3 tablespoons) of chilled unsalted butter, cubed

125mL (½ cup) of buttermilk

⅔ cup (150 grams) of mashed pumpkin

Extra buttermilk for glazing

1. Place a shelf in the middle of your oven before preheating to a temperature of 200°C/390°F.

2. Into a large mixing bowl add the flours, baking powder, cinnamon, nutmeg, sugar and salt. Mix the dry ingredients together and then add the butter. Using your fingertips rub the butter into the flour mixture until it resembles fine breadcrumbs.

3. Make a well in the centre of the mixture and add the buttermilk and pumpkin. Use a flat-bladed knife to bring the mixture together before turning it out onto a lightly floured surface. Gently knead the dough until it just becomes smooth.

4. Roll the dough out to a thickness of about 2cm (1 inch) and then use a 6cm (2 inch) scone cutter to cut out the scones. Bring the remaining dough together and reroll it to cut out the remaining scones.

5. Line a baking try with baking paper and then place the scones onto the tray so they are just touching. Use a pastry brush to glaze the scones with some of the extra buttermilk before placing them into the preheated oven.

6. The scones will take around 12 to 15 minutes to cook and will have a lovely golden top and when tapped on the bottom will sound hollow.

7. Eat the scones while they are still warm out of the oven and wrap them in a tea towel to prevent them from drying out.

Quail egg bites with bacon and chives

I am frequently asked to bring along a plate of these bite-sized sensations when I'm invited to a cocktail party or even an afternoon tea. The salty bacon and the freshness of the chives create a beautiful pairing for the tender quail eggs.

24 quail eggs

120mL (⅗ cup) of thickened (heavy) cream

150 (5.3 ounces) of bacon finely diced

Salt and pepper

3 tablespoons of snipped chives

1. Place a shelf in the middle of your oven before preheating to a temperature of 200°C/390°F.

2. Grease a 24 hole mini muffin tin and set it aside until required.

3. Place the diced bacon into a heavy based frying pan and cook over medium heat until browned and slightly crispy.

4. Remove the pan from the heat and place a teaspoon of bacon into the bottom of each muffin hole.

5. Crack a quail egg into each muffin hole before adding a teaspoon of cream. Use the handle of the teaspoon to carefully jiggle the contents of each bite to roughly combine the cream, egg whites and bacon pieces while being careful to keep the yolk whole.

6. Crack some freshly ground black pepper over the top along with a sprinkling of salt and the snipped chives.

7. Place the tin in the preheated oven for around 10 minutes until the tops of the bites are slightly browned and the egg is set.

8. Set the tin aside for 5 minutes before carefully removing the bites and serving them while still warm from the oven. You can make these ahead of time as they are beautiful at room temperature.

Onion jam tartlets with goat's cheese

— MAKES 24 —

These beautifully 'short' tartlet shells provide the perfect accompaniment to the deliciously sweet and slightly tangy onion jam. Beautiful fresh goat's cheese crumbled over the top just before serving provides the final touch.

PASTRY

130 grams (1 cup) of super-fine white rice flour

70 grams (¾ cup) of glutinous rice flour

110 grams (4 ounces) of cold unsalted butter, cubed

Pinch of salt

40 - 60mL (2 - 3 tablespoons) of cold water

ONION JAM

500 grams (1 pound) of Spanish (red) onions, peeled, halved and finely sliced

Extra virgin olive oil

Salt and pepper

75mL (⅓ cup) of red wine

30mL (1½ tablespoons) of balsamic vinegar

1½ tablespoons of white wine vinegar

60 grams (3 tablespoons) of light muscovado sugar

125 grams (4.4 ounces) of fresh goat's cheese

1. Place the flours, butter and salt in the bowl of your food processor and pulse until the mixture resembles bread crumbs. Slowly add the cold water until the dough comes together and forms a ball.

2. Remove the dough from the food processor and roll it out between two sheets of baking paper to a thickness of around 3mm (⅛ inch).

3. Butter your tartlet trays to ensure the shells do not stick. Check your pastry cutter to ensure you have the right size and then cut out the shells. Gently ease the shells into the tartlet molds and re-roll the pastry to cut out the remainder.

4. Once you have prepared all the tartlet shells cover them in glad wrap and place the trays into the refrigerator while you prepare the onion jam.

5. Pour some olive oil into the bottom of a large heavy based saucepan. Heat the pan over a low to medium heat before you add the onions, a pinch of salt and some pepper. Cook the onions for about 30 minutes until they soften and become translucent. You will need to keep an eye on them and stir occasionally to ensure they don't stick. The onions need to cook slowly and gently to release their natural sugars, which will create the beautiful, luscious caramel flavours in the jam.

6. Bring the heat up a little as you add the wine and vinegars and give the mixture a stir to ensure everything is combined. Bring the mixture to the boil and then turn it down so it is just simmering and add the sugar. Continue to cook on a low heat until most of the liquid has evaporated — this will take around another 30 to 40 minutes. Remember to stir occasionally as it would be such a shame for it to catch and burn after all your hard work.

7. Once the liquid has mostly evaporated remove the pan from the heat and set aside to cool.

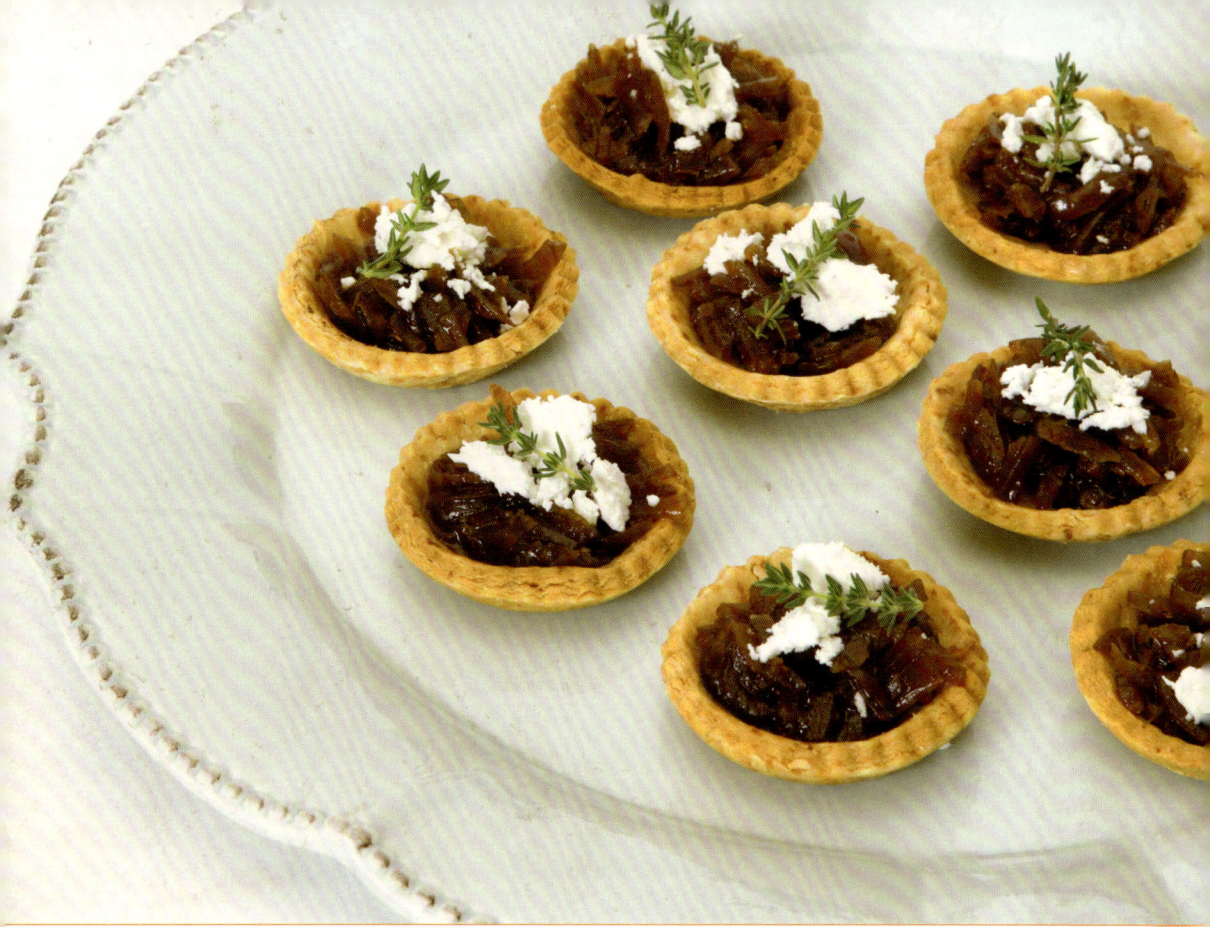

8. Place a shelf in the middle of your oven before preheating to a temperature of 180°C/356°F.

9. Remove your tartlet shells from the refrigerator and after removing the glad wrap place them in the preheated oven and bake for around 10 minutes until they are just starting to colour. Remove the tartlet shells from the oven and place a teaspoon of onion jam into each before returning them to the oven for another 5 minutes to allow the onion jam to bubble and the pastry to finish cooking and turn a lovely golden colour.

10. Once the tartlets are ready remove them from the oven and crumble a little goat's cheese over the top of each one before serving.

11. Any extra onion jam will keep in a jar in the refrigerator for about a month. If you pre-prepare your pastry shells you can have them sitting in the freezer so if friends drop by unexpectedly you can pop them straight in the oven from the freezer, add the jam and you've got a tasty morsel for everyone to enjoy.

Mini lamb meatballs with pinenuts and currants

— MAKES 40 —

These Moroccan inspired meatballs are a great start to any party and with the tahini and yoghurt dipping sauce provide both warmth from the spices and cool and savoury yoghurt with fresh bursts of coriander.

MEATBALLS

100 grams (3.5 ounces) of pinenuts

Extra virgin olive oil

1 onion finely chopped

500 grams (1 pound) of lamb mince

100 grams (3.5 ounces) of currants

Zest and juice of a lemon

1 teaspoon of ground coriander

1 teaspoon of ground cumin

½ teaspoon of ground cinnamon

½ teaspoon of ground clove

4 tablespoons of finely chopped parsley

Salt and pepper

DIPPING SAUCE

2 tablespoons of tahini

200 grams (⅔ cup) of yoghurt

Large handful of coriander finely chopped

Juice of half a lemon

1. Place a shelf in the middle of your oven before preheating to a temperature of 200°C/390°F. Line two baking trays with baking paper and set them aside while you prepare the meatball mixture.

2. Place the pinenuts into a small heavy-based frying pan and dry roast them over a medium heat being careful to keep them moving as the natural oils will be released and they will colour quickly. Once the pinenuts have a lovely golden hue, remove them from the heat and place in a small bowl to cool.

3. Add a little olive oil to the already heated frying pan and add the chopped onion. Gently sauté the onion until it softens and takes on a slightly golden translucency. Once the onions are cooked, remove them from the heat and place them in a small bowl to cool.

4. Place all of the ingredients into a large mixing bowl including the now cooled pinenuts. Add salt and pepper to taste, being sure to add a little more than you might think the mixture needs. Use your hands to bring the mixture together. Be quite thorough when you combine the mixture so all the ingredients are evenly distributed and the mixture sticks together.

5. Form the mixture into small balls of about 3cm (1 inch) in diameter and place them on the lined baking trays.

6. Place the trays of meatballs into the oven to bake for 15 minutes until the balls are golden brown and still slightly pink in the middle.

7. While the meatballs are cooking place the tahini, yoghurt, coriander and lemon juice into a bowl and mix until well combined.

8. Once the meatballs are cooked remove them from the oven and place them in a serving bowl with some toothpicks and the dipping sauce.

Cucumber bites with smoked salmon

— MAKES 30 —

The slices of cucumber make for such a refreshingly delightful crunch and a wonderful accompaniment to the oiliness of great quality smoked salmon. Horseradish adds a peppery heat that complements the crème fraiche.

2 Lebanese (or small) cucumbers

150 grams (5.3 ounces) of smoked salmon slices

100 grams (⅓ cup) of crème fraiche

1 tablespoon (20 grams) of lilliput (extra fine) capers roughly chopped

Zest of a lemon finely chopped

1 tablespoon of chervil finely chopped

Salt and pepper

2 tablespoons of horseradish cream

30 chervil sprigs for garnish

1. Slice the cucumbers into rounds of about 7mm (½ inch) thick and arrange them on your serving platter. Place the crème fraiche into a bowl along with the capers, lemon zest and chervil and mix to combine. Check for seasoning and add some salt and pepper if needed.

2. Place a teaspoon of the crème fraiche onto each cucumber round and top it with a piece of smoked salmon. I like to drape the salmon over the cucumber so that it creates a beautiful nest that has some height but also accentuates the round shape of the bite.

3. On top of the smoked salmon place a dollop of horseradish cream and finish it off with a sprig of chervil.

4. You can prepare these bites ahead of time and keep them fresh in the refrigerator until you're ready to serve them.

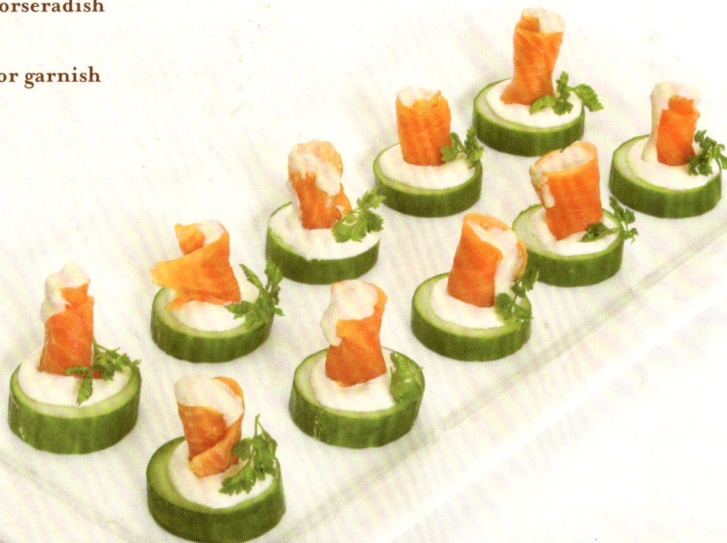

Cannellini bean dip
with crudités

Some friends had called and I invited them over for a few drinks that afternoon. I had beautiful fresh vegetables as I'd been to see Robbie at the farmer's market that morning and I thought hummus would be a great accompaniment. I adore hummus — the nuttiness of the tahini and the bursts of lemon and garlic make for a dip worthy of its cult status. Upon examination of the pantry I discovered that I didn't have any chickpeas but did have some wonderful organic cannellini beans so thought I'd give them a go as a substitute. I loved the result — it was so creamy and subtle. This recipe has evolved over time and the parsley adds wonderful freshness.

240 grams (8.5 ounces) of dried cannellini beans

I teaspoon of bicarbonate of soda

1.6 litres (6 cups) of water

260 grams (I cup plus 2 tablespoons) of tahini

6 tablespoons of lemon juice

4 cloves of garlic crushed

6 tablespoons of roughly chopped parsley

6 tablespoons of cold water

Salt

A selection of crudités such as carrot sticks, radishes, cauliflower, red capsicum slices and snow peas.

I. Place the cannellini beans in a large bowl and cover them with cold water — the beans will expand as they rehydrate so be sure to add twice as much water as you have beans. Set the beans aside to soak overnight. Dried beans can take quite some time to cook and for a dip you need them to be extremely soft. I went to school with an Egyptian girl and her mother showed me this trick to help them soften and cook more quickly.

2. The following day, drain the beans and place them in a saucepan over a high heat along with the bicarbonate of soda. Stir the beans for a couple of minutes over the heat before pouring in the cold water. Bring the water to the boil and let the beans simmer for around 20 minutes until soft and starting to break up a little.

3. Drain the beans well before adding them to your food processor and giving them a good blitz until you have a smooth paste. Keep the processor going while you add the tahini, lemon juice, garlic and parsley so they are incorporated evenly. Add about a teaspoon of salt before slowly adding the cold water which will help make the dip a little smoother and also lighter. Keep mixing the dip for another few minutes as this will ensure you have an extremely creamy result.

4. Once you are happy with the consistency, taste and adjust the seasoning before placing the dip in your serving bowl and setting it aside to allow the flavours to mingle for about half an hour before serving.

Entrees

MY HUSBAND is a wonderful violinist. He has played since he was six years old and is one of the most versatile players I know — whether he's performing a violin concerto or sonata, ripping out an improvised break out with his indie rock band or having a jam with a Klezmer ensemble, he loves it all.

Music has been an important part of our lives; in fact the first time I saw Jeremy was when he was the soloist for Vaughan Williams' most beautiful of pieces: The Lark Ascending. I still played the violin in those days and his playing took my breath away — he has such a sweet sound.

Needless to say, music has continued to be an ongoing feature in our lives, and for our tenth wedding anniversary a few years ago we decided to combine four of our mutual loves: Paris, food, music and the 1920s by holding a 1920s Parisian themed party complete with Gypsy swing band.

Now, being somewhat of a perfectionist I'll admit to becoming a little obsessive with the preparations — to the point that I almost tipped my darling husband out of the car one Sunday afternoon when we drove past an amazing swing band busking at a local shopping street. The good news is that we ended up hiring the band for the night and they were indeed brilliant, so maybe it was worth Jeremy's near-death experience…

When cooking for a large party you really want to have a mixture of hot and cold hors d'oeuvre but also ensure you don't end up spending the entire night preparing food. The best way to achieve this balance is to think about what you can prepare ahead of time and up to what stage. It may be that for some things you can have them all-but-done and waiting covered in plastic (cling) wrap in a cupboard or the refrigerator. For other items you may be able to have them ready and waiting to go straight into the oven when your guests start arriving. The most important thing to do is fully plan out the menu — this way you'll give yourself the best chance to have a relaxing and enjoyable evening (really, most of us want to be home entertainers, not caterers!).

On this particular night we served a vast array of small bites. Gougères, crudités with hummus and roasted capsicum dip, onion jam tartlets, chicken liver pate, smoked salmon on fresh baguette slices with cream cheese and dill. Mini lamb meatballs were part of our savoury selection along with a wonderful selection of French cheeses, which we laid out on our large chopping block with bunches of dried muscatels.

The dessert course included mini morello cherry cupcakes with sour cream icing, delicate and fragrant apricot and sauvignon blanc jellies, chocolate and strawberry roulade and the piece de resistance: my very first golden towering croquembouche.

The Gypsy swing band played and Jeremy of course joined in for a jam, friends arrived with dresses of fringe and dinner suits, wearing headbands and posing with their long cigarette holders. It was an incredible night and everyone commented on the beautiful food. Most of the people in the room were eaters of gluten and they all had a wonderful night with not an ounce of gluten being consumed (and without anyone even noticing).

Cream of chestnut soup

— SERVES 6 —

This soup has a wonderfully fragrant and delicate flavour and is the perfect starter for any dinner party. The texture of the chestnuts creates a velvety soup while the larger pieces give a lovely textural element. I think this is the perfect beginning for a Christmas celebration as it is quite light but helps ease everyone into a festive mood.

700 gram (1.5 pound) tin of whole chestnuts

30 grams (1 ounce) of unsalted butter

1 large onion, finely chopped

3 stalks of celery, finely chopped

1 litre (4 cups) of chicken or vegetable stock

Salt and pepper

500mL (2 cups) of milk

Parsley finely chopped for garnish

1. Place a large saucepan over a low heat and add the butter. Once the butter has melted add the onion and celery and sauté until soft and translucent. Add the chestnuts along with the stock and season with salt and pepper. Bring the stock to the boil with the lid on and reduce the heat to maintain a slow simmer for 10 minutes.

2. I find the best utensil to crush the chestnuts is a potato masher as it allows you to crush some of the chestnuts till quite smooth and others are left in larger pieces. Once you have crushed the chestnuts add the milk and stir to combine as this will ensure the liquid doesn't split. Bring the soup back to a simmer for another 10 minutes while you chop up the parsley.

3. Serve the soup in individual bowls and scatter the parsley over the top just prior to serving.

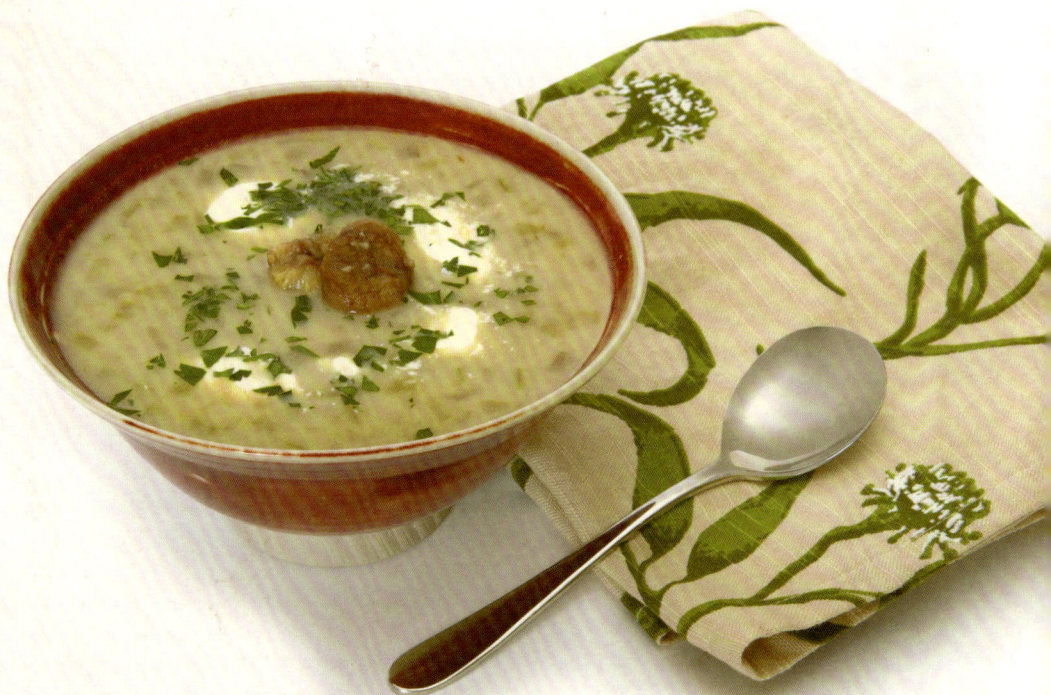

Crêpes with a creamy mushroom filling

— SERVES 8 —

The brandy and paprika with the earthy mushrooms and sweet leeks makes for a wonderful looking and smelling filling; and what dish isn't enhanced by the addition of a sprinkling of gruyere?

CRÊPES

3 large egg yolks

37mL (1½ cups) of milk

65 grams (½ cup) of super-fine white rice flour

35 grams (¼ cup) of glutinous rice flour

30 grams (2 tablespoons) of brown rice flour

60mL (3 tablespoons) of brandy

100mL (5 tablespoons) of melted butter

Extra melted butter for the pan

FILLING

30 grams (1 ounce) of butter

1 large leek thinly sliced

3 cloves of garlic crushed

10 grams (2 tablespoons) of rice flour

700 grams (25 ounces) of Swiss brown mushrooms thinly sliced

2 tablespoons of brandy

375mL (1½ cups) of thickened cream

150 grams (5.3 ounces) of grated gruyere cheese

4 tablespoons of parsley finely chopped

Salt and pepper

1. Place a shelf in the middle of your oven before preheating to a temperature of 170°C/340°F. Grease a deep baking dish with butter and set it aside while you prepare the crêpes.

2. Sift the flours into a medium mixing bowl and stir to combine. Make a well in the centre of the flour mixture and add the egg yolks, milk and brandy. Using a balloon whisk combine the ingredients until they form a smooth batter. Add the melted butter and whisk again to combine. The consistency of the batter should be similar to that of thickened cream.

3. Heat your crêpe pan over a medium to high heat and brush with a little of the extra melted butter. With a ladle place enough batter into the pan to form a delicately thin crêpe. I tend to pour the batter onto one side of the pan and as I pour I start to tip and swirl the pan so that the bottom is covered in a consistently thin layer.

4. Let the crêpe cook for a minute or two until the bottom is a lovely golden colour and then use an egg flip to turn and cook the other side for another minute.

5. Place the crêpe on a plate lined with paper towel and remember to brush the pan with a little melted butter before you add the batter for the next crêpe. Finish making all the crêpes (you should have 12) and then cover the plate of crêpes with a tea (dish) towel to keep them moist while you prepare the filling.

6. Place a large heavy based frying pan over a medium heat and add the butter. Once the butter has melted add the leek and garlic and sauté with a little salt until the leek is soft and tender.

7. Once the leeks are ready add the flour to the pan and stir for about a minute to allow the flour to start cooking out. Now add the mushrooms and some more salt and let the mushrooms cook down for about 10 minutes until you have lovely slightly golden soft mushrooms.

8. Pour the cream into the pan and stir to combine the ingredients. Bring the cream up to the boil and let it simmer for a few minutes until slightly thickened.

9. Remove the pan from the heat and add the parsley. Stir the parsley through the mixture and then set the pan aside to cool. Once the mushroom mixture has cooled to room temperature you are ready to fill the crêpes.

10. Take the first crêpe and place it flat on the bench in front of you. Spoon four tablespoons of the mushroom mixture in the centre of the crêpe and then use the back of the spoon to spread the mixture over the crêpe leaving a 2cm (1 inch) border around the edge.

11. Take some of the gruyère cheese and sprinkle it down the centre of the crêpe in a line. Now roll the crêpe up into a log shape and place it in the greased baking dish. Repeat the process with the remaining crêpes until you have a baking dish filled with lovely mushroom filled crêpes.

12. Spoon any remaining mushroom sauce over the top of the crêpes and then grate over some extra gruyère cheese.

13. Cover the dish with aluminium foil being careful to ensure the foil isn't touching the crêpes as the cheese will stick as it melts.

14. Place the dish in the preheated oven and let the crêpes cook for around 20 minutes before removing the foil and allowing the top to turn a lovely golden colour. This will probably take another 10 minutes.

15. Serve the crêpes with a few salad leaves and a final sprinkling of parsley.

Tarragon scallops wrapped in prosciutto with celeriac puree

— SERVES 6 —

Whenever anyone mentions scallops my mouth starts watering as I think about the sweet tender meat that, each time tasted, seems to be even more succulent than remembered. In this recipe I couple the sweetness of the scallops with salty prosciutto and the subtle fragrance of celeriac — the ugliest looking vegetable I have ever seen. The bumpy, lumpy skin is cut away to reveal beautiful white flesh that when steamed and blended makes a fantastically smooth puree.

2 celeriacs (celery root)

18 scallops

9 slices of prosciutto

4 tablespoons of fresh tarragon leaves

Salt and pepper

Extra virgin olive oil

Juice of two lemons

6 tarragon sprigs for garnish

1. Peel the celeriac by cutting just below the skin — the outer edge is quite firm and dense so be sure to cut it away so the flesh cooks evenly. Chop the celeriac into pieces — maybe eighths and place them into a saucepan. Cover the celeriac pieces with water and add a little salt before placing the pan on the heat and bringing it to the boil. Turn the heat down and let them simmer until tender — around 15 minutes.

2. While the celeriac is simmering you can start to prepare the scallops. Place the tarragon leaves in a bowl, such as a mortar, and add some salt and pepper. Grind up the leaves until you have a paste and then add a few tablespoons of olive oil and stir to combine.

3. Remove the scallops and prosciutto from the refrigerator and cut each slice of prosciutto in half lengthways. Rub the tarragon paste all over the scallops and then wrap each one in a slice of prosciutto and use a toothpick to hold it in place.

4. Your celeriac should be ready, so drain it well and place the pieces into the bowl of your food processor along with some salt and pepper. Turn on the processor and slowly add some olive oil as the puree becomes smooth and creamy. Taste for seasoning and leave while you cook the scallops.

5. Place a large heavy based frying pan on a high heat and once hot place the scallops in the pan. Sear the scallops for around 2 minutes on each side — the prosciutto will crisp up and keep the tender scallops moist and succulent. Remove the scallops from the pan and carefully take out the toothpicks.

6. Place the celeriac puree in the middle of each plate and then top each plate with three scallops. The scallop pan should still be warm so deglaze it with the lemon juice and then pour these juices over the scallops. Serve with a sprig of tarragon for garnish.

Venetian inspired soup

— SERVES 6 —

My husband and I had left Paris very early to fly to Venice. It was September and the acqua alta meant that Piazza San Marco was only accessible via a labyrinth of duckboards which we needed to traverse, with our hefty luggage in tow, to reach our apartment. By the time we were settled it was mid-afternoon and we hadn't eaten since breakfast. We sat at a table in one of the many Venetian alleyways and I had a soup that was so pleasingly satisfying that when I arrived home I spent quite some time trying to recreate that soup. This recipe is my interpretation of that delicious mid-afternoon meal.

60mL (3 tablespoons) of extra virgin olive oil

2 medium onions finely chopped

2 sticks of celery finely diced

3 rashers of bacon finely diced

300 grams (10.6 ounces) of tomatoes roughly chopped

300 grams (10.6 ounces) of green lentils

8 cups (2 litres) of beef stock

5 tablespoons of grated parmesan cheese

30 grams (1 ounce) of butter cut up into small cubes

Salt and pepper

Parsley finely chopped for garnishing

1. Place a large heavy based pot over a medium heat and add the olive oil. Add the onion and celery to the pot and keep moving to allow it to soften without adding too much colour.

2. Once the vegetables are soft add the bacon and cook for a further 2 minutes to allow the bacon to start to render.

3. Add the tomatoes, lentils and stock to the pot and bring it to the boil before reducing the heat so you maintain a slow simmer. Place the lid on the pot and allow the soup to simmer until the lentils are tender. This will take around 30 minutes but may take longer depending on the age of the lentils.

4. Once the lentils are cooked, taste the soup and season with a little salt and lots of freshly ground black pepper. Don't add too much salt as the parmesan will contribute to the salt content and you can always add a little more later if you feel it needs adjusting.

5. Take the pot off the heat and whisk in the butter and parmesan cheese. Taste the soup one last time and adjust the seasoning as required before serving it with a sprinkling of parsley.

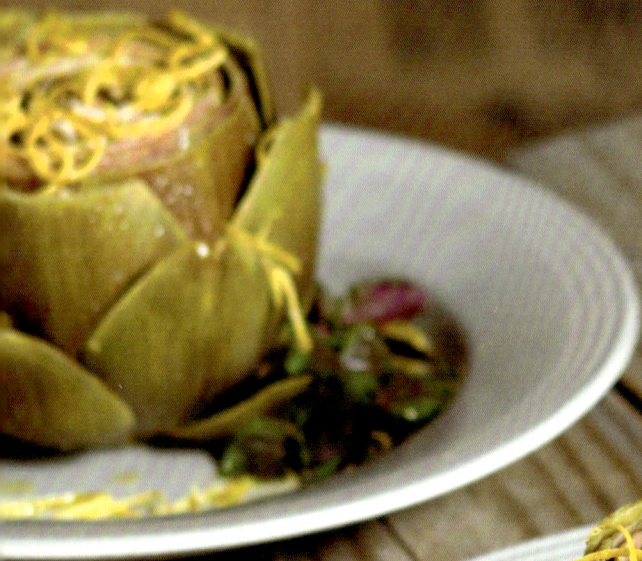

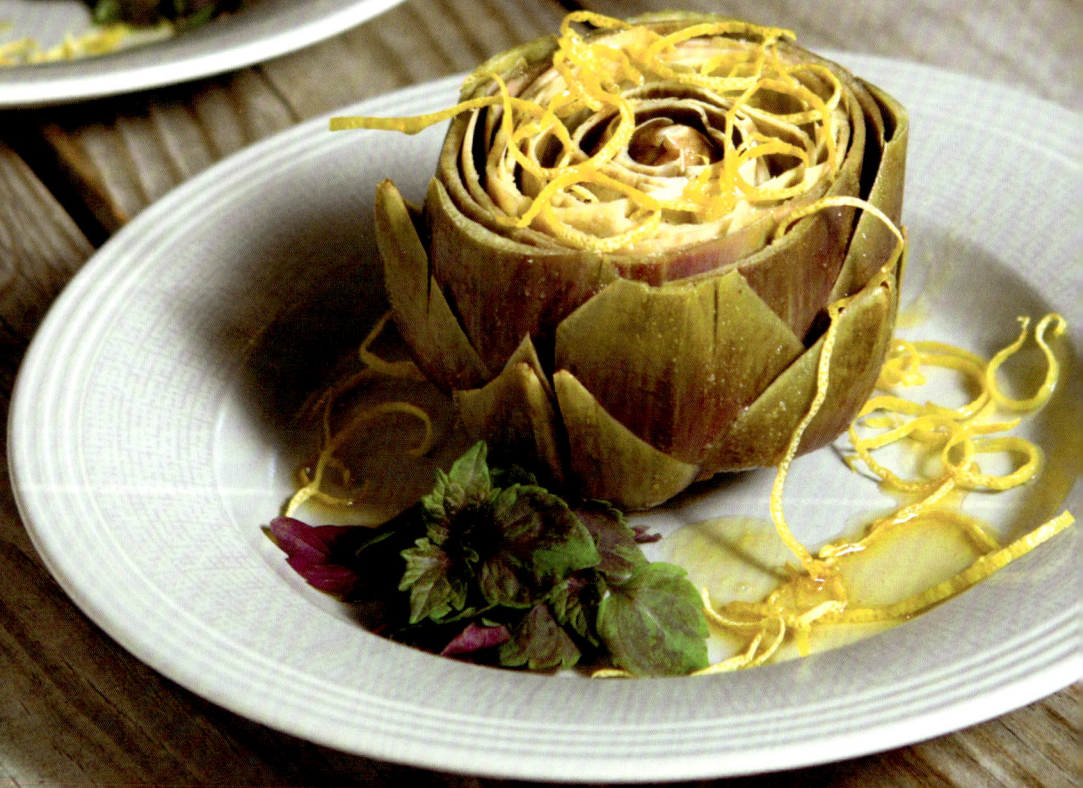

Artichokes with lemon scented butter

— SERVES 6 —

Artichokes are one of those vegetables that people seem to shy away from due to those terrifying stories of hours spent in the kitchen trimming, removing the choke and oxidation from the air resulting in a less-than-appetizing dish. This is a very simple way to prepare and enjoy these most special of vegetables.

6 large globe artichokes

2 large lemons

150 grams (⅔ cup) of butter

1. Remove the zest from the lemons and set this aside until later. Now cut the lemons into quarters.

2. Fill up your kettle and bring the water to the boil.

3. Cut the stalk off from the base of each artichoke and trim the base of the flower so that it sits flat. Now cut about the first third of the flower off the top – around 2 - 3cm (1 inch).

4. Rub and squeeze the lemon juice over all the cut areas of the artichokes to prevent the flesh from oxidising.

5. Arrange the artichokes in a heavy based pan that is large enough for them to fit in a single layer with their cut leaves facing up. Pour over the boiling water so the artichokes are covered and throw in the lemon pieces. Place a plate on top of the artichokes to keep them submerged before placing the lid on the pan.

6. Simmer the artichokes for around 20 minutes or until you can easily insert a knife tip into the base of the artichokes.

7. Remove the artichokes from the water and allow them to drain on some paper towel while you prepare the sauce.

8. Place a small saucepan over a medium heat and add the butter and lemon zest. Allow the butter to colour until it is a lovely nutty brown and then remove it from the heat.

9. To serve this dish simply place an artichoke in the centre of each plate and open up the outer leaves slightly before drizzling over the lemon scented melted butter.

10. Serve immediately and be sure to encourage your guests to use their hands to gently prise each leaf away, dip it in the melted butter before dragging it across their teeth to remove the edible flesh. As you get closer to the heart of the artichoke you will be able to eat the entire leaf before removing the choke and eating the sweetest part of an artichoke – that beautiful heart.

Lamb fillets with pickled cucumber salad

— SERVES 6 —

I love to serve this as an entrée for a summer dinner party. The still crisp and lightly pickled cucumber provides lovely freshness alongside the meltingly tender lamb fillets. A squeeze of lemon and a dollop of yoghurt provide the final flourish.

LAMB FILLETS

1 teaspoon of ground cumin

1 teaspoon of ground coriander

1 teaspoon of sweet paprika

½ teaspoon of cayenne pepper

Salt and pepper

600 grams (21 ounces) of lamb fillets

PICKLED CUCUMBER

4 Lebanese (or small) cucumbers

½ a medium Spanish (red) onion

65mL (¼ cup) of white wine vinegar

10 grams (2 teaspoons) of golden caster sugar

Salt and pepper

TO SERVE

150 grams (⅔ cup) of plain yoghurt

1 lemon cut into quarters

4 tablespoons of coriander (cilantro) finely chopped

1. To prepare the lamb fillets, place the spices into a plastic bag along with some salt and pepper. Hold the bag closed and give the spices a shake to form an even mix. Add the lamb fillets and keep the bag closed so you can toss the lamb fillets in the spice mix until they are coated all over. Set the lamb aside while you prepare the cucumbers.

2. Slice the cucumbers into thin rounds. Cut the onion into quarters and then finely slice it before placing the onion and cucumber slices into a bowl.

3. Add the vinegar, sugar and a little salt and pepper to the vegetables and give everything a good stir so each slice of cucumber is coated in the vinegar mixture. Set the vegetable aside while you cook the lamb fillets.

4. Pour a few tablespoons of olive oil into the plastic bag with the lamb fillets and massage it around to evenly coat each piece of meat.

5. Heat a griddle pan over a high heat and place the lamb fillets on the hot pan. Cook the fillets for three minutes on each side before removing them from the pan and setting them to rest for three more minutes.

6. To serve the dish place a circle of cucumber and onion slices in the centre of each plate. Cut the rested lamb into angled slices of around 1cm (½ inch) in thickness and create a mound of these on top of the cucumber. Add a dollop of yoghurt on top of the lamb and a lemon wedge on the side of each plate. Add a sprinkle of coriander and serve immediately.

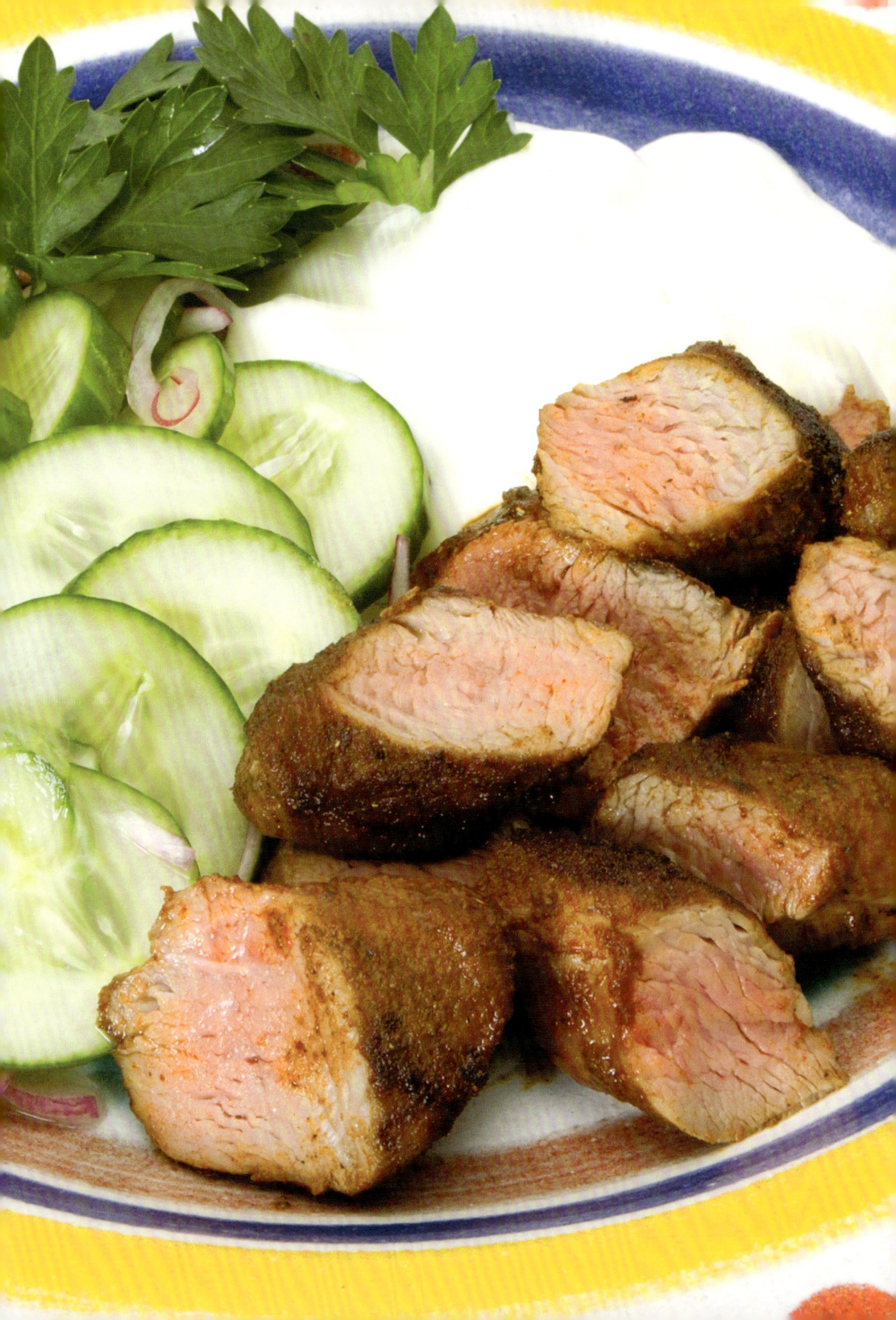

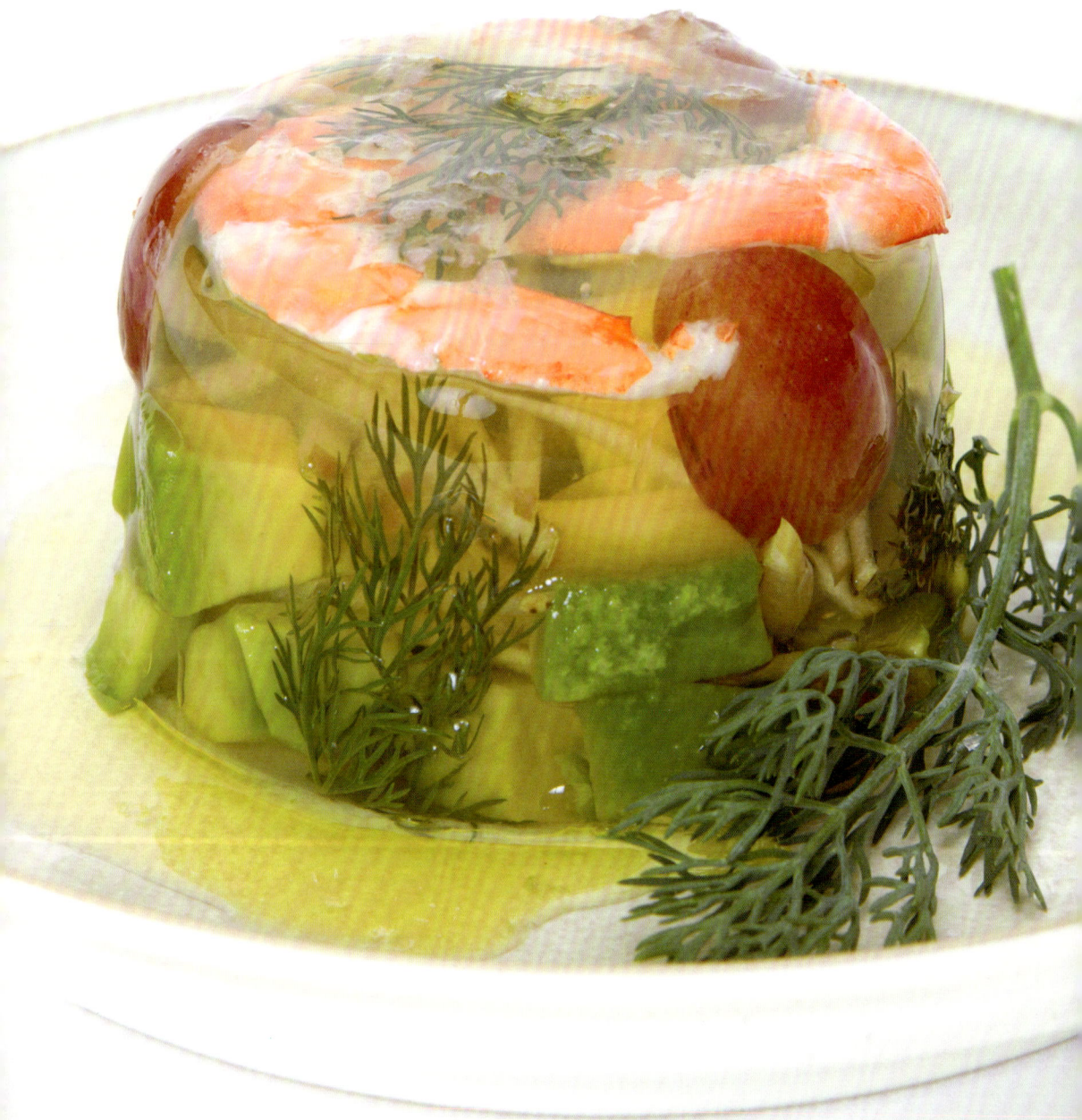

Apple, grape, avocado and prawn jellies

— SERVES 6 —

Maggie Beer introduced me to the delights of verjuice and its tremendous versatility through her wonderful television series The Cook and the Chef. *In this recipe I took the idea of a prawn cocktail, and instead of the traditional heavy mayonnaise of the 1970s version, I have encased it in a delightfully gentle verjuice jelly. This dish is so simple yet provides the desired 'wow factor' when delivered to the table.*

375mL (1½ cups) of verjuice

20 grams (1 tablespoon) of golden caster sugar

A few stems of dill plus 18 small sprigs

2½ leaves of gelatin (2 grams or 0.07 ounces each)

9 medium sized cooked prawns (shrimp) cut in half lengthways

1 large avocado cut into 1cm (½ inch) dice

½ a crisp apple such as a pink lady cut into matchsticks

9 red flame grapes cut in half lengthways

Extra virgin olive oil

1. Pour the verjuice into a small saucepan along with the sugar and place it over a medium heat to bring it to the boil. As soon as the liquid reaches boiling point turn off the heat and add the dill stems to steep for five minutes before removing them from the liquid.

2. Place the gelatin leaves into a bowl of cold water and allow them to soften for around five minutes before squeezing out the excess liquid and adding them to the verjuice. Stir the mixture until the gelatin disappears before setting the saucepan aside to allow the mixture to cool to room temperature.

3. Take six small ramekins and arrange the avocado, apple and grapes, keeping the presentation in mind for when you tip the jellies out. Take three prawn halves and push them around the sides of the ramekins and then do the same with the dill sprigs.

4. Pour the now cooled verjuice into the ramekins then cover them in cling film and place them in the refrigerator for at least a couple of hours.

5. When you are ready to serve the jellies place the ramekins into a bowl of hot water for a few seconds and then tip them upside down onto the centre of your serving plates. Drizzle a little olive oil over the top and finish with a sprig of dill just before serving.

Salad of orange with olives and fennel

— SERVES 6 —

This is a lovely and fresh start to a summer dinner party. As always, simplicity mandates the need for the best of ingredients. Make this when you happen upon the ripest of oranges — Valencias are perfect with their sweet flesh and lovely golden orange colour. I like to use two different kinds of oranges if I have the luxury as the flavours and colours add additional contrast to the dish.

2 Valencia and 2 blood oranges

2 baby fennel bulbs

18 small black olives

100 grams (3.5 ounces) of Persian feta

Extra virgin olive oil

Salt and pepper

1. Peel the oranges following the contour of the fruit and being sure to remove all the bitter pith. Slice the oranges into thin rounds.

2. Arrange three slices of orange on each entrée plate if serving as individual portions or covering the base of a large platter to serve in the middle of the table. Sprinkle the orange slices with a little salt and a good amount of freshly ground pepper.

3. Remove the tops from the fennel bulbs and set the fronds aside to use as a garnish. Cut the base from the fennel bulbs and then slice the fennel into paper thin vertical slices and scatter these over the orange.

4. Arrange the olives attractively and then crumble the Persian feta into the centre of the salad.

5. Sprinkle a little more salt and pepper and then scatter over the roughly torn fennel fronds. Finish with a drizzle of olive oil just as the dish is served.

Main Courses

NOT EVERYONE LOVES TO COOK and not everyone has the confidence to grab some ingredients and throw together a dish. Some people love the process of perfecting the recreation of a recipe and seeing how close they can get to the photograph in the cook book. Others enjoy reading recipes and gathering ideas and drawing on these when creating their dishes.

I form part of the latter group – it is rare for me to adhere to a recipe, so the process of writing this book has been an adventure in and of itself.

My usual cooking style is to think about the sort of dish I would like to create and then plan from there. If preparing a main course I will start with the core ingredient, which will usually be a meat protein. From here I will consider the cut of meat and the most appropriate way for it to be cooked. For example if I were preparing a shoulder of hogget (meat from a sheep that is between one and two years of age) then the connective tissue and marbled fat need long slow cooking to render, become tender and fall away from the bone. A lean cut such as a backstrap of beef is best cooked quickly to retain moisture and cooked to medium rare.

Once I have thought about how I'd like to cook the cut then I turn to the flavour profile – do I want a rich winter warmer or a lighter summery style? Do I want flavours of Provence with its thyme, rosemary and olive oil or maybe a Moroccan profile of coriander and cumin seeds, preserved lemon and sour cherries?

Texture is a very important element of a dish and without it the flavour is lost. This also needs to be considered when preparing a meal and may take the form of the side dishes to accompany a main course or maybe the garnish of an entrée. A scattering of toasted nuts in a salad may add that final crunch that takes it from a good salad to something really interesting and exciting to eat.

These decisions help me formulate the final dish in my head and from there I understand the processes I will need to undertake, the utensils and pans I will need and whether the stove top, oven or grill will be the provider of heat.

This approach allows me to cook confidently without the need to religiously adhere to a recipe. Now this approach does come with its successes and failures but I find that the more I follow this process of exploration the more confident I become, and the better I understand how ingredients respond when cooked in different methods and also when paired with other flavours.

The recipes in this book are the result of much trial and error and refinement but this does not mean that they are written in stone. I encourage you to take these ideas and adapt them to create variations and new ideas that can feed into your cooking.

Roasted pumpkin, spinach and pinenut lasagne

— SERVES 8 —

This is a great dish to prepare ahead of time and then simply slip into the oven to bake. The caramelised onions and golden pinenuts make a great addition to the roasted pumpkin and the centre layer of spinach and ricotta provides a more traditional element to the dish.

1 whole butternut pumpkin (squash)

4 onions

4 large sprigs of rosemary

260 grams (9.2 ounces) of pinenuts

Extra virgin olive oil

Salt and pepper

Nutmeg

1 large bunch of spinach

400 grams (14 ounces) of ricotta cheese

400 gram (14 ounce) tin of diced tomatoes

1 large ball of mozzarella cheese

500 grams (17.6 ounces) gluten free lasagne sheets

1. Place two shelves near the middle of your oven before preheating to a temperature of 180°C/355°F. Line two baking trays with baking paper and set them aside while you prepare the vegetables.

2. Cut the pumpkin into 2cm (1 inch) cubes and do the same with the onions. Distribute the vegetables evenly between the two baking trays and then scatter with the rosemary leaves and pinenuts. Season with salt and pepper before drizzling with olive oil and massage the pumpkin pieces so they are evenly coated.

3. Place the trays into your preheated oven and let the pumpkin and onion roast until they are golden and caramelised. This will take around 20 minutes.

4. While the pumpkin is roasting you can prepare the spinach and ricotta layer. Chop up the spinach leaves and steam them for 2 minutes until they have just wilted. Place the spinach into a large mixing bowl and add the ricotta cheese. Season with salt and pepper, grate in some nutmeg and then use a fork to break up the ricotta and combine the spinach.

5. I like to place the lasagne sheets into a bowl of hot water for a couple of minutes before I place them in the dish but read the instructions on the packet to ensure you prepare them correctly.

6. Into the bottom of your lasagne dish place the pumpkin and onion mixture from one of the baking trays. Top this with a layer of lasagne sheets before spreading the spinach and ricotta over the pasta in an even layer. Follow this with another layer of lasagne sheets before the remaining roasted pumpkin and onion. Add a final layer of pasta before pouring the tin of diced tomatoes over the top. Cut the mozzarella ball into slices and lay these over the top of the tomatoes. Your lasagne is now ready to bake.

7. Place the dish into the preheated oven and let it bake for 40 to 60 minutes. Check if the pasta is cooked by inserting a knife into the centre of the dish — it should be easy to insert with little to no resistance. Once the pasta is cooked, and the mozzarella has turned a wonderful golden colour, remove the lasagne from the oven.

8. The lasagne will be incredibly hot so leave it to sit for 10 minutes. This will make it easier to serve and provides you with time to prepare a crisp green salad to accompany this delicious dish.

I often prepare this dish and take it with us when staying in a holiday house with friends. It makes for a tasty and simple first night dinner accompanied by a green salad.

Perch with a caper, lemon and white wine sauce

— SERVES 2 —

I love to use orange roughy for this dish — the flesh is so delicate and the fish has such a lovely sweetness that matches beautifully with the salty capers and the acidity from the lemon and wine.

Extra virgin olive oil

4 fillets of perch

2 shallots (eschallots) finely sliced

2 tablespoons of lilliput (extra fine) capers

Juice of a lemon

100mL (3.38 fluid ounces) of white wine

30 grams (1 ounce) of butter

Salt and pepper

1. Place a large heavy-based frying pan onto a medium to high heat and add a little olive oil. Season the fillets with salt and pepper and then place them into the hot pan with their skin side down.

2. The fillets will only need to cook for two to three minutes on each side. When the second side is cooked remove the fish from the pan and place the fillets onto the serving plates to rest while you prepare the quick sauce.

3. Into the hot pan add a little more olive oil if needed before sautéing the shallot slices for a couple of minutes. Once the shallots have softened add the capers and wine to the pan. Let the wine reduce down to a few tablespoons before pouring in the lemon juice.

4. Once the liquid returns to the boil add the butter and keep it moving around the pan so it incorporates into the liquid to form the sauce.

5. Pour the lemon and white wine sauce over the fillets and serve immediately.

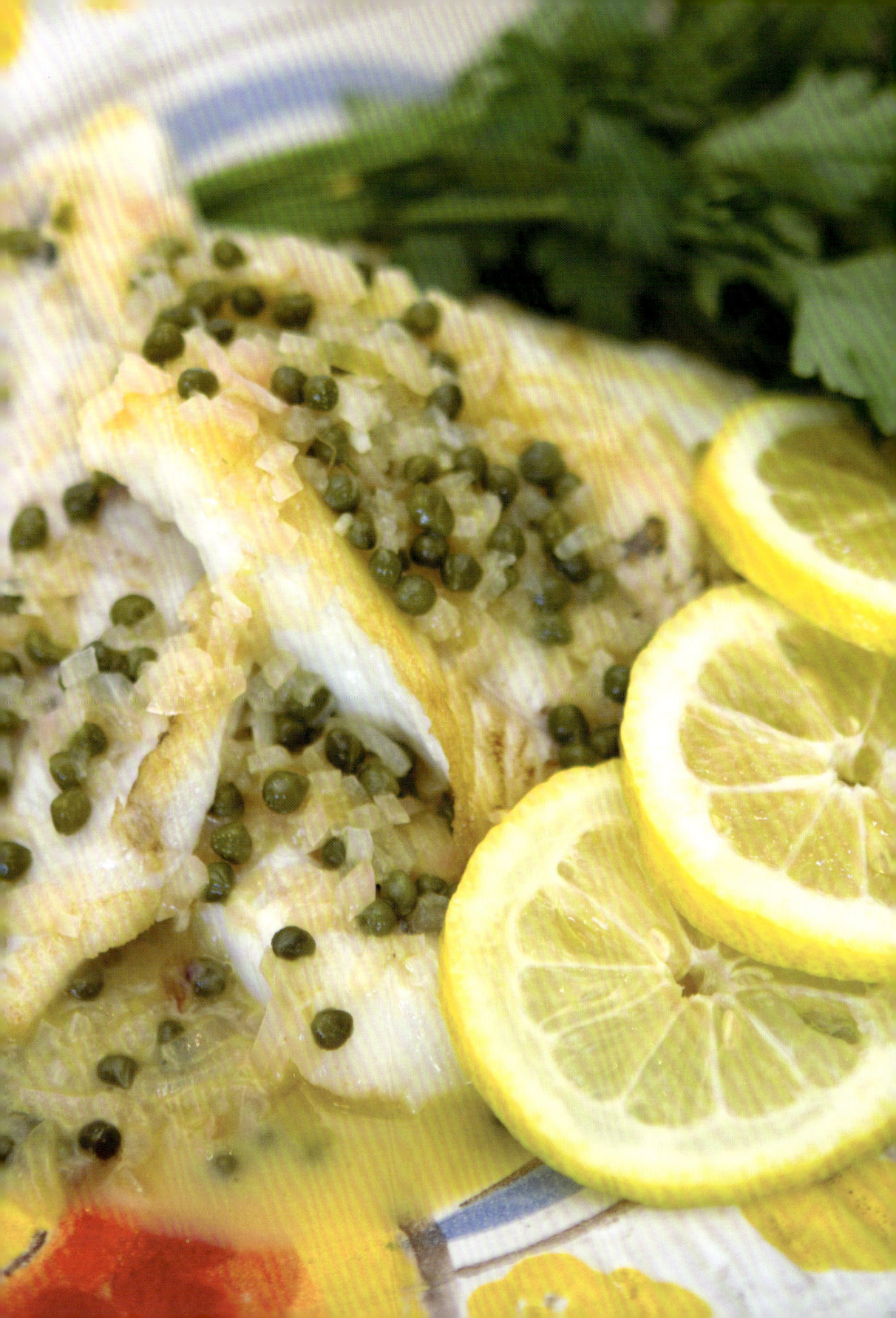

Spaghetti with meatballs in a tomato sauce

— SERVES 8—

As a child, coming home from school to learn that we were having spaghetti for dinner was… disheartening. Gluten free pasta was terrible and extremely expensive so while my siblings enjoyed their long strands of spaghetti I ate my Bolognese sauce on top of steamed rice. How wonderful it was when quality gluten free pasta became available and I could enjoy those strands of spaghetti I had wanted so much to eat as a child.

MEATBALLS

Extra virgin olive oil

2 large onions finely chopped

2 cloves of garlic crushed

500 grams (1.1 pounds) of pork mince

500 grams (1.1 pounds) of veal mince

4 tablespoons of parsley finely chopped

Salt and pepper

SAUCE

1 large onion finely chopped

2 cloves of garlic crushed

4 rashers of bacon cut into lardons

400 gram (14 ounce) tin of diced tomatoes

700mL (23.6 fluid ounces) jar of passata (tomato puree)

4 tablespoons of oregano finely chopped

2 tablespoons of parsley finely chopped

Salt and pepper

1. In a large heavy based pot add two tablespoons of olive oil and once heated add the onions and garlic for the meatballs. Sprinkle some salt to help bring out the juices and stir the onions as they soften. Once the onions are well softened and translucent remove them from the pot and place them in a large mixing bowl.

2. Add the parsley and some salt and pepper to the onions and stir the ingredients together before adding the pork and veal mince. Use your hands to incorporate the onions and herbs through the meat. Keep mixing the meat through your hands until it becomes slightly sticky.

3. Once the mince is ready, roll it into balls around 3cm (1.2 inches) in diameter and set them aside while you prepare the tomato sauce.

4. Place the same heavy based pot you used to soften the onions for the meatballs over a medium heat and add a little more olive oil. Once it has heated up add the onions and garlic for the sauce and again stir these along with some salt until they soften and become translucent.

5. Once the onions have softened add the bacon lardons and sauté them until browned and slightly crisp.

6. Pour in the tinned tomatoes and the passata along with the chopped oregano and parsley. Stir the sauce until everything is combined.

7. Bring the sauce to the boil and then add the meatballs. Bring the sauce back to the boil and turn the heat down to low so it gently simmers. Place the lid on the pot and leave it to simmer for an hour.

8. Once the sauce has finished simmering, check the seasoning and adjust accordingly.

9. Serve the sauce on top of or mixed through your favourite spaghetti and sprinkle with some freshly grated parmesan cheese just before serving.

Whole baked trout with lemon and thyme

— SERVES 6 —

A friend took my husband and me trout fishing a few times and all I can say about fishing is that it clearly has nothing to do with catching fish. You spend the day working your way up a river or around a lake and at the end of it you have… nothing. Thank goodness I can go to my fishmonger and buy a few of these stunning looking and tasting fish.

6 trout each weighing around 450 grams (15.9 ounces) (ask your fishmonger to gut and scale for you)

2 bunches of thyme

Salt and pepper

Extra virgin olive oil

3 lemons

1. Place a shelf in the middle of your oven before preheating to a temperature of 240°C/465°F. Line a baking tray with baking paper and set it aside while you prepare the trout.

2. Remove the leaves from a bunch of thyme and place them in a bowl along with a good lug of olive oil and big pinch of salt and some freshly ground black pepper. Mix this together and then rub this all over the fish — inside and out.

3. Split the other bunch of thyme into sixths and place a bunch inside the cavity of each fish before placing them on the oven tray.

4. Cut the lemons in half and then cut the ends off each half so that the lemon sits flat. Nestle the lemon halves in and around the trout before placing the tray into your hot oven.

5. The fish should take around 10 to 12 minutes to cook. You can check they are ready by sticking a knife into the thickest part of one of the fish and seeing if you can easily lift the flesh away from the bone.

6. Once the fish are cooked remove the tray from the oven and place a fish and a baked lemon half onto each plate.

7. Simple sides are the answer for this dish — maybe some green beans with toasted almonds along with some boiled potatoes.

8. Peel the skin of the fish back to reveal the wonderfully succulent mushroom pink flesh and then squeeze over the juice from the baked lemon before tucking into what is an often overlooked fish.

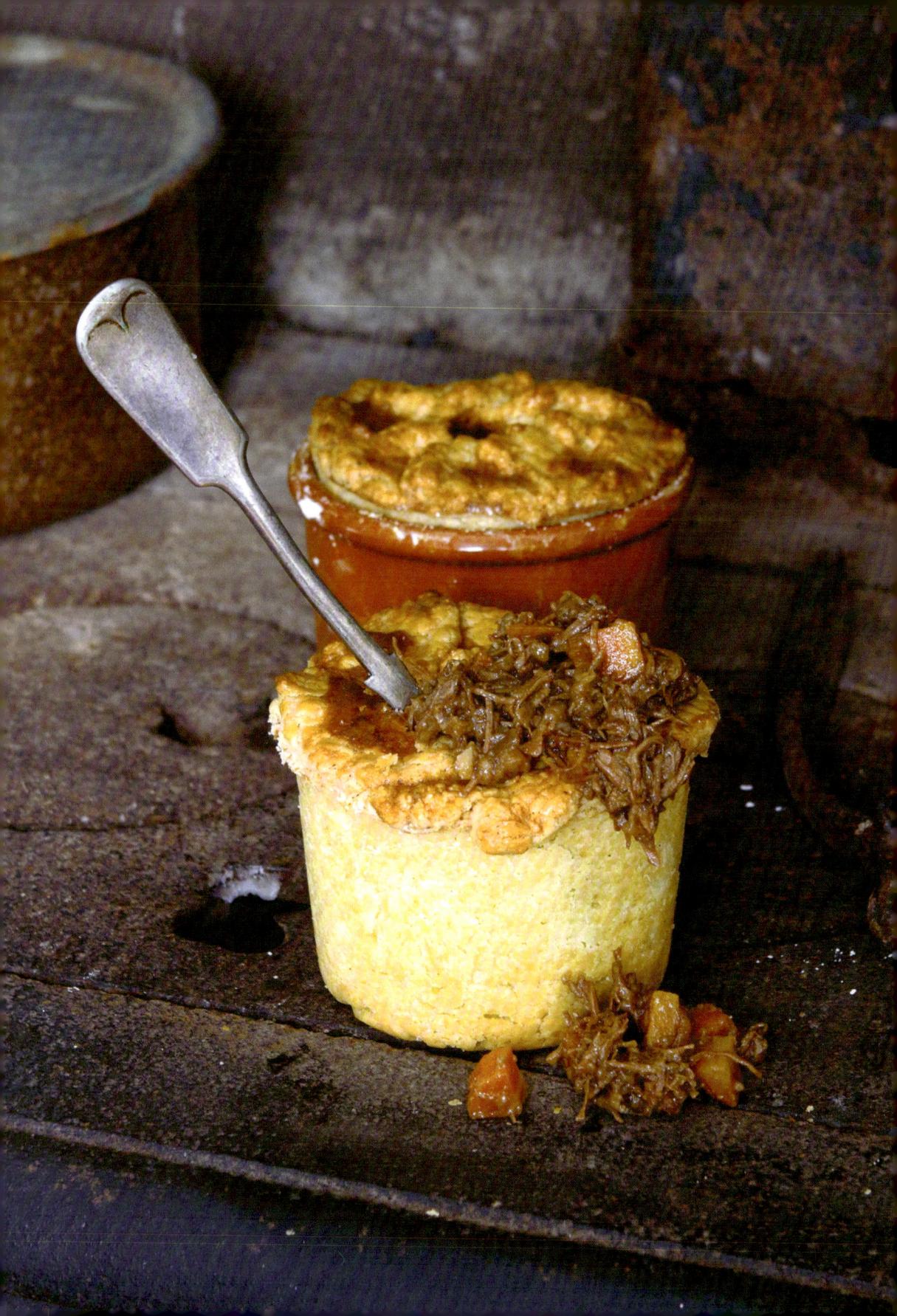

Beef and ale pie

— SERVES 4 —

When my husband and I took our first trip to London our first stop was the local pub where Jeremy proceeded to order with glee a pint of winter ale and a beef pie. The pastry looked so short and crisp and I sat there while he enjoyed his foodie moment and wondered how I could replicate his bliss back home. After some trial and error the following recipe received Jeremy's seal of approval.

PASTRY

200 grams (7 ounces) of butter

165 grams (1¼ cups) of super-fine white rice flour

85 grams (⅔ cup) of glutinous rice flour

125mL (½ cup) of sour cream

FILLING

Extra virgin olive oil

1 kilogram (2.2 pounds) of oyster blade steak cut into 3cm (1.2 inches) chunks

Salt and pepper

3 tablespoons of super-fine white rice flour

1 large onion finely diced

3 cloves of garlic crushed

2 carrots cut into cubes

700mL (23.6 fluid ounces) of gluten free beer

A bouquet garni of thyme, parsley stalks, a celery stick and bay leaves

250mL (1 cup) of beef stock

20mL (1 tablespoon) of red wine vinegar

20 grams (1 tablespoon) of dark muscovado sugar

1 egg lightly whisked for glazing

1. The first thing to start on is the pie filling as this will need stewing time during which you can prepare your pastry.

2. Place the chunks of beef into a plastic bag along with some salt and pepper and the 3 tablespoons of rice flour. Hold the bag closed and toss the meat through the flour until it evenly coats each piece of beef.

3. Place a large heavy-based pot over a high heat and add a couple of tablespoons of olive oil. Once the pan has reached temperature add some of the flour-dusted beef pieces being careful not to over-crowd the pan. Brown the meat well on all sides and then remove it to a plate to start on the next batch of beef. You will probably need to do this in three to four batches to ensure the meat browns well and seals rather than stews which will happen if you place too much meat into the pot.

4. Once all the meat has been browned and has been set aside on the plate you can now commence sautéing the vegetables. Add the onion, garlic and carrot to the pot and reduce to a medium heat. Stir the vegetables as they soften in the oil for around 5 minutes.

5. Return the beef to the pot and add the beer, bouquet garni, stock, vinegar and sugar.

6. Bring the stew to a boil and reduce the heat to low so it maintains a very slow simmer. Place the lid on the pot and leave it to simmer for three hours being sure to check it occasionally and ensure it isn't catching on the bottom of the pot.

7. Taste the stew and adjust the seasoning accordingly — it will likely need some more salt and pepper as you have not added any except for the seasoning of the flour.

8. Remove the pieces of beef from the stew and use two forks to shred the meat. Don't shred it too finely as you still want to have some texture of the meat pieces in the final pie. Remove the bouquet garni from the stewing liquid before adding the shredded meat back into the pot. Stir the meat through the stew and check the seasoning for a final time before turning off the heat and leaving it to cool to room temperature. It's important that you allow the stew to cool completely otherwise you will melt the pastry when you add the mixture into the cases. While it's cooling down you can prepare the pastry.

9. Place a shelf in the middle of your oven before preheating to a temperature of 200°C/390°F. Take four 250mL (1 cup) ramekins and place them on a baking sheet and set them aside while you prepare the pastry dough.

10. Into the bowl of an electric mixer add the butter and sifted flours. On a low speed mix until combined, increasing the speed as the mixture starts to come together. Add the sour cream and again mix to combine, starting slowly and increasing speed as the dough stabilises.

11. Roll out two-thirds of the dough to a thickness of about 3 millimetres and then cut out four circles, each one large enough to cover the bottom and sides of your ramekins. Place the pastry circles into the ramekins and shape them accordingly. The pastry is quite a soft dough so if you tear it or make a hole you should be able to easily fill it in with a little extra pastry.

12. Roll out the remaining pastry dough and cut out four circles, just larger than the top of your ramekins.

13. Divide your cooled stew between the four pastry lined ramekins, which should be filled almost to the top.

14. Place a pastry lid onto each pie and press the edges together to ensure you have a seal all the way around each pie. Trim off any excess pastry and then with a sharp knife cut a small slit in the centre of each pastry crust. This will allow excess steam to escape while the pies are baking.

15. Brush the top of each pie with the whisked egg to help the pies develop a lovely golden crust before placing the tray of pies into the pre-heated oven. The pies will need to bake for 30 minutes to ensure the pastry is cooked through and the top has turned an inviting golden colour.

16. Once the pies are cooked remove them from the oven and leave to sit for 10 minutes before removing them from their ramekins and serving along with a crisp garden salad.

Oven baked ratatouille

— SERVES 6 —

Ratatouille is one of those dishes that always exceeds my expectations. As with any dish the key to success is the quality of the ingredients but for me the simple flavours of ratatouille make this rule more important than usual. For this reason the thought of summer instantly generates thoughts of sitting in the sunshine with a bowl of ratatouille and a glass of rosé.

2 large eggplants (aubergines)

4 zucchini (courgettes)

3 red capsicums (bell peppers)

4 Roma (egg) tomatoes

2 large brown onions

4 cloves of garlic crushed

A bunch of basil

Salt and pepper

Extra virgin olive oil

1. Place a shelf in the middle of your oven before preheating to a temperature of 200°C/390°F.

2. Cut up the eggplants, zucchini, capsicums, tomatoes and onions into 2.5cm (1 inch) cubes and place them into a baking dish. Add the crushed garlic and the roughly torn leaves of the basil keeping a couple of sprigs aside as garnish.

3. Sprinkle salt and pepper over the vegetables and then add a few good lugs of olive oil – about 5 to 6 tablespoons.

4. I find the easiest way to coat the vegetables in the oil is to use my hands to gently toss the vegetables together.

5. Once the vegetables are evenly coated in the oil cover the dish with foil and place it in the preheated oven.

6. The ratatouille will take around an hour to cook but give it a stir a couple of times to make sure everything is cooking evenly.

7. Once the ratatouille is ready the eggplant will impart a lovely creaminess to the dish and the vegetables will still hold their shape but will give easily when pushed with a spoon.

8. Serve the ratatouille in bowls with a sprig of basil for garnish and a slice of good bread to mop up the juices.

Braised pork chops with lemon and prunes

— SERVES 4 —

This is a lovely simple dish to prepare with the final result of big flavours and a beautiful sauce belying the simplicity. I love to serve this with some creamy mashed potatoes and lightly sautéed kale.

Extra virgin olive oil

4 pork loin chops

Salt and pepper

6 shallots (eschallots) finely sliced

8 sage leaves

60mL (3 tablespoons) of brandy

250mL (1 cup) of white wine

250mL (1 cup) of veal stock

12 pitted prunes (dried plums)

Juice of two lemons

30 grams (1 ounce) of butter

1. Pour a couple of tablespoons of olive oil into a heavy based large saucepan. Season the pork chops with salt and pepper before browning them over a high heat in the olive oil.

2. Once the pork has browned on both sides remove the chops to a plate and add the shallot slices to the pan. Sauté the shallots for a couple of minutes so they soften and start to release their sweet flavour before adding the finely sliced sage leaves and allowing them to sauté for a minute.

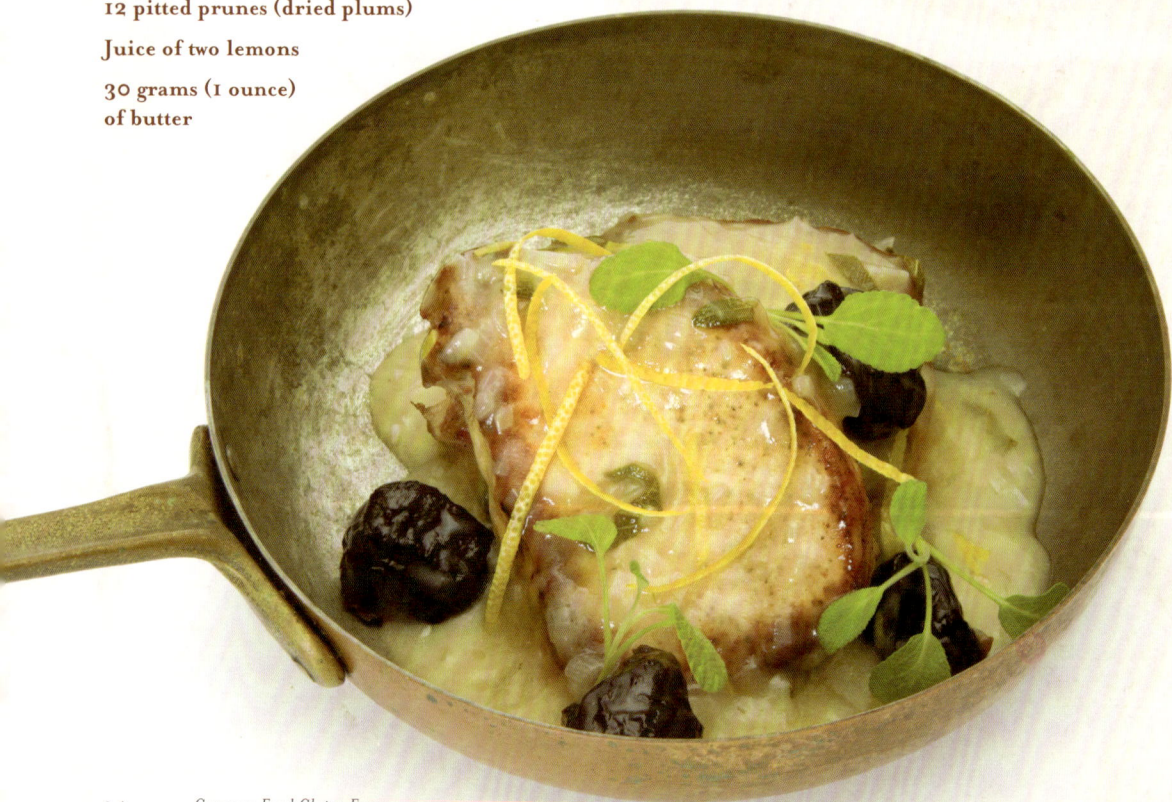

3. Return the pork to the pan and add the brandy. Allow the alcohol to cook off from the brandy for a minute before adding the white wine. Once the wine has come to the boil add the veal stock and bring the liquid back to the boil.

4. Turn the heat to low to maintain a slow simmer before scattering the pitted prunes into the pot and nestling them between the pork chops.

5. Pour in the lemon juice and place the lid on the pan and leave it to simmer gently for 20 minutes.

6. Remove the pork and prunes from the liquid and turn the heat to high so the liquid boils rapidly. Allow the sauce to reduce by half and thicken slightly. Remove the pan from the heat and add the butter stirring constantly so it emulsifies into the liquid. Give the sauce a taste and adjust the seasoning accordingly.

7. Return the pork and prunes to the sauce and turn them over so they are coated. Now serve the chops along with the prunes and some of that beautiful lemon and sage sauce.

Tarragon roast chicken marylands with gravy

— SERVES 6 —

This is a great recipe to make for two or three when you want the majesty of a Sunday roast but don't need to cook a whole bird or joint of meat. Tarragon is a herb that isn't used often in home cooking but it is probably my favourite of all herbs. It has a wonderful subtle anise flavour, which is the perfect accompaniment for naturally reared, free-range chicken.

CHICKEN

6 chicken marylands with their skin on

120 grams (½ cup) of softened unsalted butter

4 tablespoons of tarragon leaves roughly chopped

Zest of two lemons

Salt and pepper

GRAVY

500mL (2 cups) of chicken stock

3 sprigs of tarragon

Juice of a lemon

Salt and pepper

40 grams (2 tablespoons) of super-fine white rice flour

60mL (3 tablespoons) of cold water

1. Place a shelf in the middle of your oven before preheating to a temperature of 220°C/430°F. Line a baking tray with baking paper and set it aside while you prepare the chicken.

2. Pour the chicken stock into a small saucepan and add the sprigs of tarragon. Place the saucepan over a high heat and bring it to the boil. Once the stock has come to the boil turn off the heat and set the pan aside to allow the tarragon to infuse through the stock.

3. Into a small bowl place the softened butter, tarragon leaves, lemon zest and a good amount of salt and pepper. Use a fork to mix the flavours through the butter so everything is well combined.

4. Wash your marylands and dry them well with some paper towel. Use your fingers to separate the skin from the meat starting at the thigh end of the joint. Try to keep the skin attached at the edges of the thigh and work your hand down to the drumstick as far as you can being careful not to break the skin.

5. Once you have loosened the skin on all the joints you are ready for the tarragon butter.

6. Take about a tablespoon of the butter in your preferred hand and with the other gently lift the skin on the first maryland. Smear the butter over the flesh of the chicken and use the skin to help push the butter down and over the drumstick. Smooth the butter over the flesh in an even layer and then smooth the skin over the top so you retain the shape. Repeat the process for each of the marylands and as you complete them arrange them on the lined baking tray.

7. Once all the marylands are ready wash your hands well and then place the tray into the preheated oven. The marylands will take approximately 30 minutes to roast (depending on their size they may take a little longer). To check that the meat is cooked insert a skewer into the thickest part of the joint and when removed the juices should run clear.

8. While the chicken is roasting you can prepare the gravy.

9. Remove the tarragon sprigs from the now cooled stock before returning the pan to the heat. Add the lemon juice and bring the stock back to the boil. Mix the rice flour and water together and add this to the stock a tablespoon at a time while stirring constantly until you achieve the desired consistency.

10. The chicken should now be cooked so remove the tray from the oven and pour the pan juices into the gravy. Set the chicken to rest while you finish preparing the gravy.

11. Stir the pan juices through the gravy until it is completely combined. The juices should thicken the gravy slightly and provide a velvety finish to the sauce. Check the seasoning and add salt and pepper as required before pouring the gravy into a gravy boat to place on the table.

12. Serve the marylands and gravy along with traditional side dishes such as roasted potatoes, pumpkin, cauliflower in cheese sauce, Brussels sprouts etc.

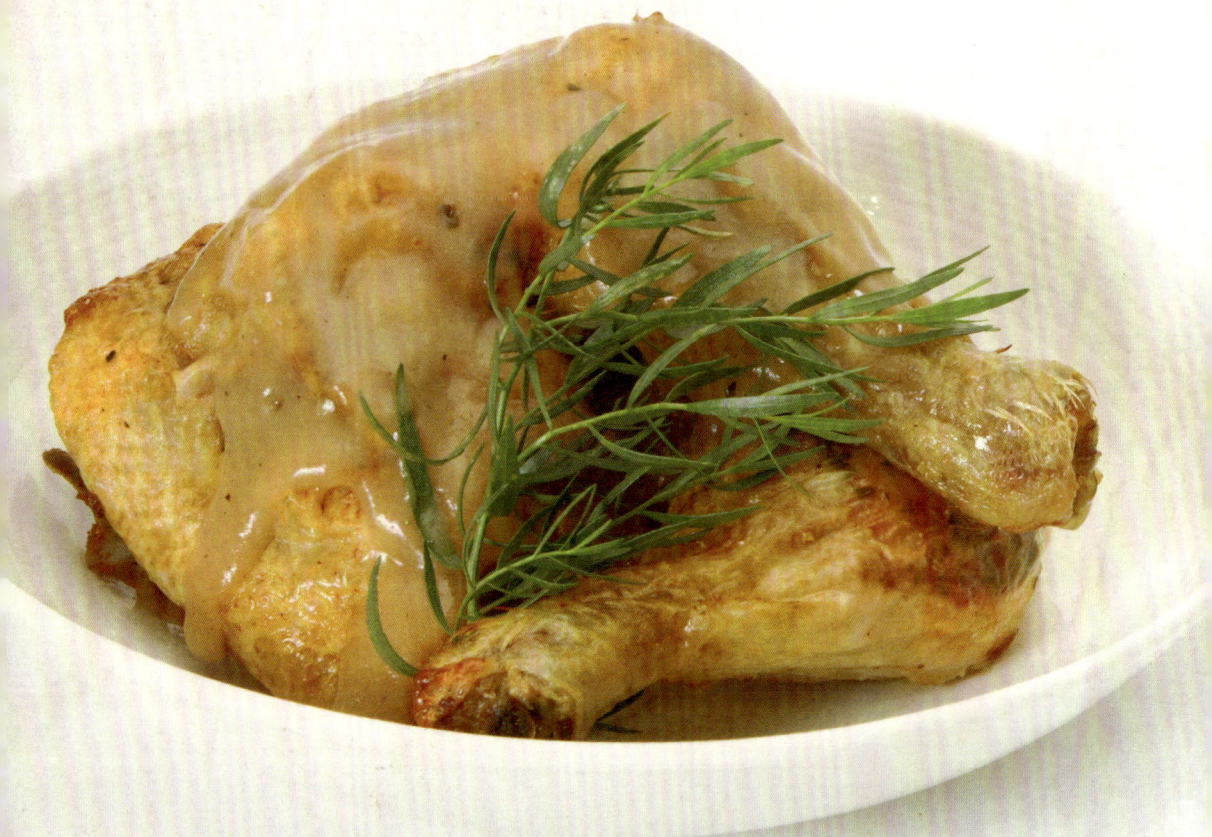

Side Dishes

WHERE DID the dinner party go?

As a child I remember my parents regularly hosting dinner parties. The guests would arrive wearing elegant evening wear and my sister and I would be allowed to stay up and chat to them while they enjoyed their apéritifs and hors d'oeuvres. Mum would often serve a pot of her chicken liver pâté and it would be my job to make the accompanying toast and cut it into squares, being sure to keep a steady supply.

They would then move into the dining room and my sister and I would head to bed, but only after polishing off any remaining pâté.

In my adult life it has been extremely rare to be invited to an actual 'dinner party'. More often than not a dinner invitation is for a barbeque, a casual bowl of pasta or maybe some homemade pizza. These are great moments and it is always such a pleasure to have someone prepare a meal for you but there is something so very special about an evening of elegant courses, beautiful wine and the fantastic company of friends.

My husband and I both work full time in pretty busy jobs so it isn't easy to find time to prepare a three or four course meal but we try to hold a dinner party a few times a year.

This usually means we spend the Saturday in the kitchen undertaking as much of the preparation as possible. We always ensure we have the hors d'oeuvres and one course completely prepared before the guests arrive — usually dessert. The other courses are also well on their way and the entrée in particular has little more than to be placed in the oven or simply plated.

This preparation means that when our guests arrive we can sit and relax with them and enjoy our apéritifs and their company without fussing around the kitchen. When we sit down to dinner I'm able to finish the preparation of the entrée and then the meal moves forward from there.

Holding a dinner party is not just about good food, wine and company it is so important to make your guests feel comfortable and have an enjoyable night. Jeremy is an incredible host; he serves drinks when our guests arrive, helps them to their seats, helps me to serve and clear plates, keeps the glasses topped up throughout the night and most importantly he makes everyone relaxed through his humour and grace.

We always receive such lovely messages after a dinner party and often receive comments about this being the first dinner party guests have attended and how enthused they are to hold one themselves.

Green beans
with toasted almonds

— SERVES 6 —

Whenever we are in Paris our first dinner is more often than not at one of the beautiful cafes near the junction of Boulevard Saint-Germain, Rue de Rennes and Rue Bonaparte in the 6ᵗʰ arrondissement. My meal is always the same — confit de canard (confit duck leg) with haricot vert (green beans) and pommes sauté (roasted potatoes).

60 grams (⅔ cup) of flaked almonds

900 grams (1.98 pounds) of green beans

20 grams (0.7 ounces) of unsalted butter

1 tablespoon of extra virgin olive oil

Salt and pepper

1. Place the flaked almonds into a dry frying pan over a medium heat. Keep the almonds moving while they dry roast because they will turn quickly and burn as their natural oils are released. Once the almonds have toasted and turned golden brown remove the pan from the heat and pour the almonds into a small bowl to cool while you prepare the beans.

2. Place a large saucepan half filled with water over a high heat and bring it to the boil. While the water is coming to the boil trim the ends of the beans.

3. Once the water is boiling add a couple of large pinches of salt before sliding in the beans. Cover the pan and quickly return it to the boil before reducing the heat to maintain a steady simmer.

4. Simmer the beans for around 5 minutes or until they are just tender. Remove them from the heat and strain the water away before returning them to the dry pan.

5. Place the beans back over the low heat and add the olive oil and butter to the pan. Toss the beans around the pan until they are coated in the butter. Crack some pepper over the beans and check them for seasoning — add a little more salt if required.

6. Once the beans are ready pour them into the serving dish and sprinkle over the toasted almonds just before serving.

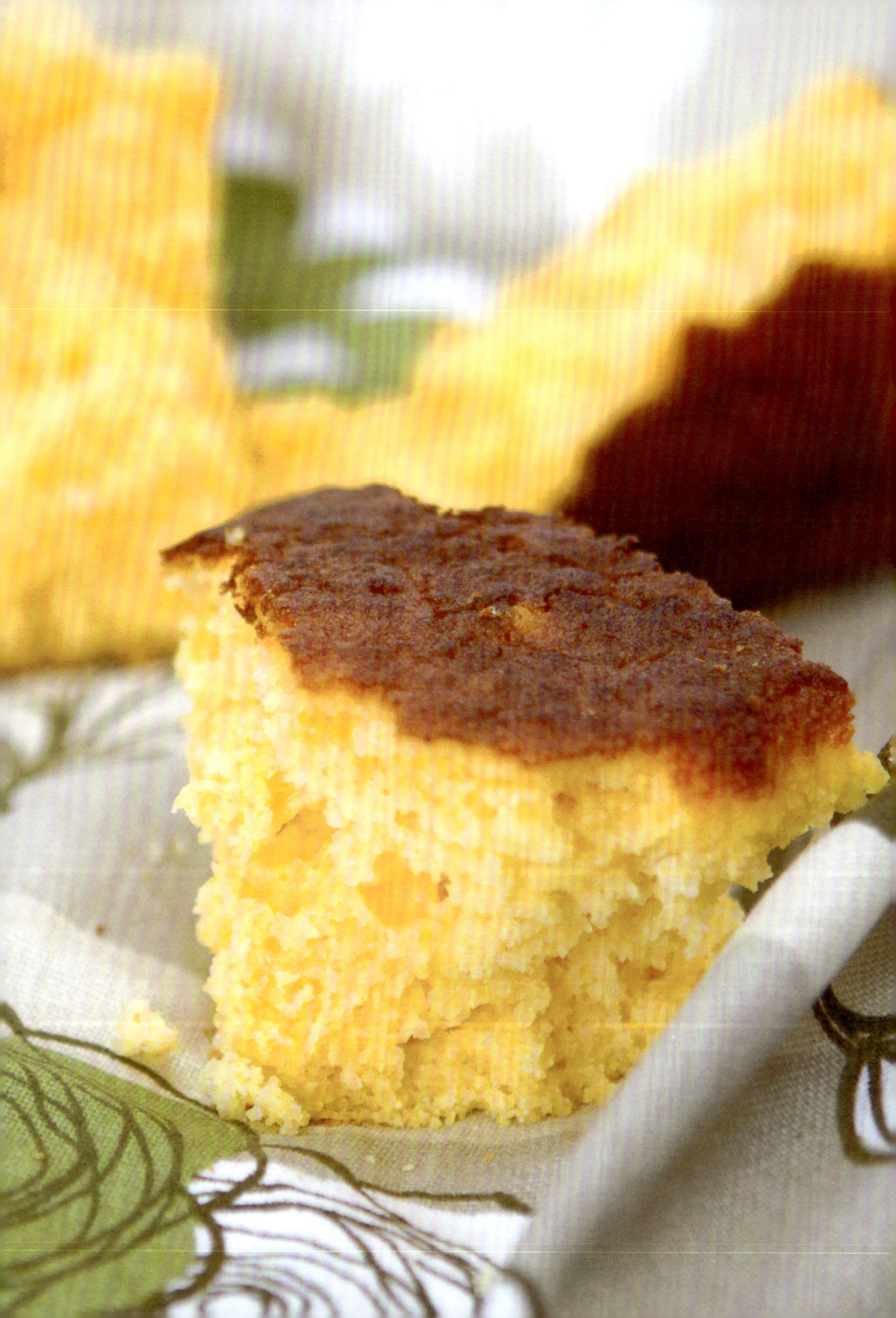

Cornbread

It's controversial but I actually love to serve cornbread with ratatouille. I find the traditional baked polenta to be a little heavy and the lighter cakelike cornbread of southern America is a perfect accompaniment to soak up the wonderful juices from the vegetables. In this recipe I use white polenta but if you can't find this then a yellow polenta will be perfectly good. Just be sure to use fine ground grain as the coarser grind creates a somewhat gritty final result. Of course this is also a perfect accompaniment to chilli con carne and other southern American dishes.

100 grams (⅔ cup) of super-fine white rice flour

50 grams (⅓ cup) of glutinous rice flour

170 grams (1 cup) of fine ground white polenta

20 grams (4 teaspoons) of gluten free baking powder

50 grams (¼ cup) of golden caster sugar

1 teaspoon of salt

250mL (1 cup) of milk

60mL (¼ cup) of vegetable oil

1 egg

1. Place a shelf in the middle of your oven before preheating to a temperature of 220°C/430°F. Grease a loaf tin with olive oil, line the base with baking paper and set it aside while you prepare the batter.

2. Place the flours, polenta, baking powder, caster sugar and salt into a large mixing bowl and stir with a wooden spoon to combine.

3. Into a jug add the milk, vegetable oil and egg. Whisk these ingredients together and then pour the mixture into the dry ingredients.

4. Use the wooden spoon to combine the ingredients to form a smooth batter.

5. Pour the batter into the greased and lined loaf tin and smooth the surface before placing it into the preheated oven.

6. The cornbread will take 25 to 30 minutes to bake and is ready when it has formed a golden crust, the edges have pulled away slightly from the inside of the tin and when inserted into the centre a skewer comes out clean.

7. Remove the cornbread from the oven and allow it to cool in the tin for five minutes before tipping it out and wrapping it in a clean tea towel. Place the wrapped cornbread onto a wire rack until ready to serve.

8. As this cornbread has a cakelike texture it won't keep particularly well as it will dry out relatively quickly. It is best served still warm from the oven but will keep for 24 hours if wrapped in plastic wrap once cold.

Ginger and orange carrots

— SERVES 6 —

Robbie Keck has a wonderful farm in Seymour, Australia, which he has developed based on the principles of biodynamic and organic horticulture. His vegetables are the best I have ever tasted, with many of them being heirloom varieties which provide great colour and flavour. His carrots are sweet and crunchy with their red skins and bright orange interiors. Orange juice brings out the natural sweetness of the carrots and ginger adds a lift for the palate which makes this dish sparkle.

900 grams (1.98 pounds) of carrots

180mL (¾ cup) of freshly squeezed orange juice

70mL (¼ cup plus 1 tablespoon) of chicken or vegetable stock

30 grams (1 ounce) of unsalted butter

2 tablespoons of ginger

Salt and pepper

1. Peel and cut the carrots into rounds about 1 inch thick and place them in a medium sized saucepan.

2. Peel the ginger and julienne it by cutting it into thin slices and then cutting these into matchsticks.

3. Add the ginger, orange juice, stock and butter along with a good pinch of salt and some freshly ground pepper to the carrots before placing the pan over a high heat and bringing it to the boil.

4. Leave the pan covered and reduce the heat to maintain a steady simmer for 4 minutes before removing the lid and allowing the liquid to continue to simmer until it completely reduces and you're left with a glaze that warmly hugs the carrots.

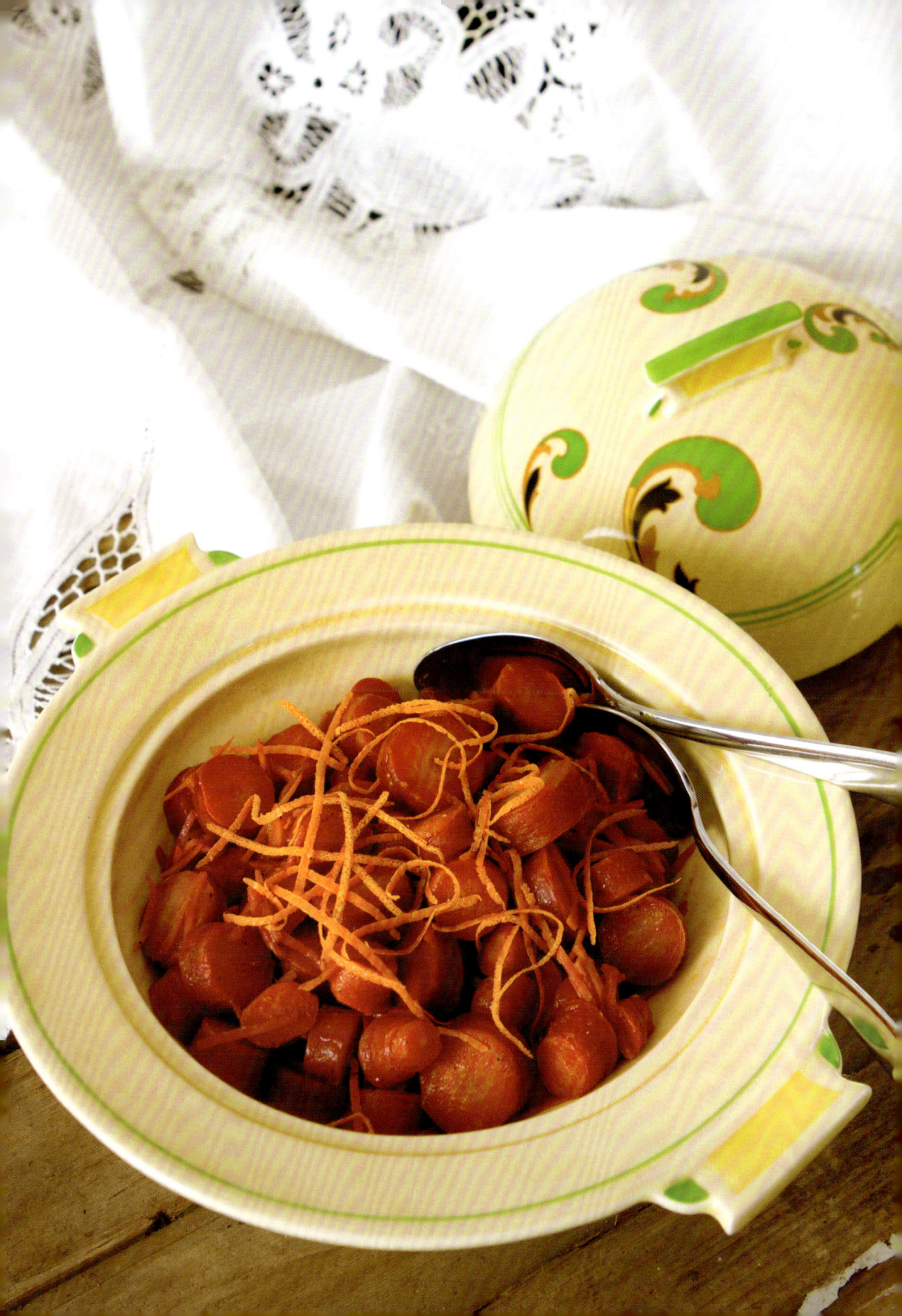

Cauliflower and cheesy Swiss chard

I think most people know and love the traditional cauliflower in cheese sauce. In this recipe I have added the earthy sweetness of Swiss chard, which adds a lovely dimension to the dish and turns this family classic into something new while still giving a generous nod to its heritage.

1 large head of cauliflower

1 bunch of Swiss chard (silverbeet)

500mL (2 cups) of milk

80 grams (⅔ cup) of super-fine white rice flour

50 grams (1.7 ounces) of unsalted butter

100 grams (3.5 ounces) of cheddar cheese grated

5 tablespoons of fresh gluten free breadcrumbs

Salt and pepper

1. Place a large saucepan half filled with water onto a high heat and bring it to the boil. Cut the cauliflower into large florets and add them to the boiling water. Reduce the heat and gently simmer the cauliflower for around 5 minutes until tender. Drain the water and cover the cauliflower with cold water. Replace the water once or twice until the cauliflower is cold and then drain it on a wire rack covered with paper towel.

2. Once the cauliflower is drained position it into a baking dish large enough to hold all the florets in a snug single layer. Set the cauliflower aside while you prepare the cheesy Swiss chard sauce.

3. Place a shelf in the middle of your oven before preheating to a temperature of 200°C/390°F.

4. Chop up the Swiss chard keeping the pieces of stalk separated from the leaves. Fill a medium sized saucepan with 6cm (2½ inches) of water and place it covered on a high heat to bring it to the boil. Once boiling, add a generous pinch of salt and add the pieces of shard stalk.

5. Simmer the chard stalks for 3 minutes and then add the leaves to the saucepan and cover. Let the chard simmer for another 2 minutes and then drain and refresh it in cold water. Set it aside and prepare the cheese sauce.

6. Return the saucepan to the heat and add the butter. Once melted and frothing add the flour and stir with a balloon whisk to form a roux. Let the roux cook out for 2 minutes stirring constantly. Pour in the cold milk while continuing to stir with the whisk. Keep whisking until the milk comes to the boil and the sauce thickens.

7. Once the sauce has thickened remove it from the heat and add the grated cheese and stir it through the sauce. Season the sauce to taste with salt and cracked black pepper and then stir through the wilted Swiss chard.

8. Pour the sauce over the cauliflower and spread it over all the florets. Sprinkle over the breadcrumbs and place the baking dish into the preheated oven.

9. Bake the cauliflower for 20 to 25 minutes until hot and the breadcrumbs have crisped up and gained some colour.

10. I like to serve the cauliflower from the baking dish at the dining table as this not only presents as a very appetising dish but also allows friends to dive in for the inevitable second helping.

Sautéed beetroot leaves

— SERVES 2 —

Most people when asked tell me that they throw the beetroot leaves away. This is such a shame as in my opinion they are just as delicious as the sweet earthy taproot. The leaves have that same sweetness found in the root of the vegetable and are accompanied by an earthy but also slightly bitter finish.

20 grams (0.7 ounce) of unsalted butter

1 tablespoon of pinenuts

1 tablespoon of currants

Beetroot leaves from a large bunch of beetroot

Salt and pepper

Juice of half a lemon

1. Place a large frying pan onto a medium heat and add the butter.

2. Once the butter has melted and started to froth add the pinenuts and allow them to toast for a couple of minutes before adding the currants.

3. Slice the beetroot leaves into thin slices and add them to the pan. Sauté them for 2 to 3 minutes or until they have wilted and become tender.

4. Season the leaves with salt and pepper, add a squeeze of lemon juice and serve immediately.

Braised cannellini beans

— SERVES 2 —

This is a great dish to make when you don't have a lot of time but want something filling and with a lovely depth of flavour. Pulses are a wonderful option as a side dish rather than the usual starches — the nutty flavour and velvety smooth texture of cannellini beans make them perfect for a braise. I usually prefer to use dried pulses but in the evening after work the convenience of tinned beans is what I need.

Extra virgin olive oil

1 large onion thinly sliced

1 clove of garlic crushed

3 sprigs of thyme

1 bay leaf

400 gram (14 ounce) tin of diced tomatoes

400 gram (14 ounce) tin of cannellini beans drained and rinsed

1 tablespoon of oregano roughly chopped

1 tablespoon of parsley roughly chopped

Salt and pepper

Juice of half a lemon

1. Heat a couple of tablespoons of olive oil over a medium heat in a deep sided frying pan. Add the sliced onion and sprinkle with a little salt to encourage the juices to release and the onion to soften without gaining much colour.

2. Once the onions have softened add the garlic and sauté for a minute before adding the thyme and bay leaf along with the tomatoes.

3. Bring the tomatoes to the boil and reduce the heat to maintain a steady simmer for 10 minutes.

4. Remove the thyme sprigs and bay leaf before adding the cannellini beans and stirring them through the tomato. Let the beans simmer for a couple of minutes to warm through before adding the chopped oregano and parsley.

5. Add a god pinch of salt and some freshly ground pepper before checking for seasoning and adjusting accordingly.

6. Squeeze in the lemon juice and stir through just before serving.

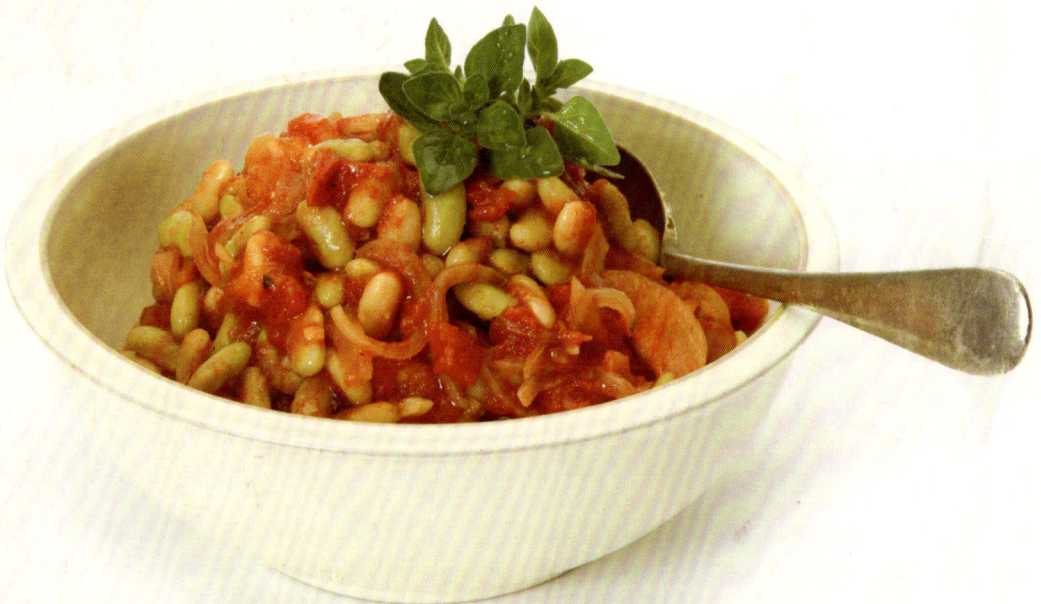

Pan-fried zucchini with garlic, mint and chilli

— SERVES 2 —

I like to use the white zucchini that actually have a beautiful variegated pale green and white skin. They tend to retain their texture and shape a little more than the usual green zucchini when cooked.

6 small white zucchini (courgettes)

Extra virgin olive oil

1 long red chilli deseeded and finely sliced

1 clove of garlic crushed

Salt and pepper

Zest of a lemon

8 mint leaves finely sliced

1. Slice the zucchini into thick rounds and set them aside while you heat the oil.

2. Into a medium sized frying pan pour a couple of tablespoons of olive oil and place the pan over a medium heat. Once the oil has heated add the sliced chilli and garlic and sauté for a minute or two until fragrant.

3. Add the slices of zucchini to the pan and toss them through the garlic and chilli flavoured oil.

4. Let the zucchini sauté for four to five minutes until the slices have softened. Sprinkle with salt and freshly cracked pepper and just before serving toss through the lemon zest and sliced mint leaves.

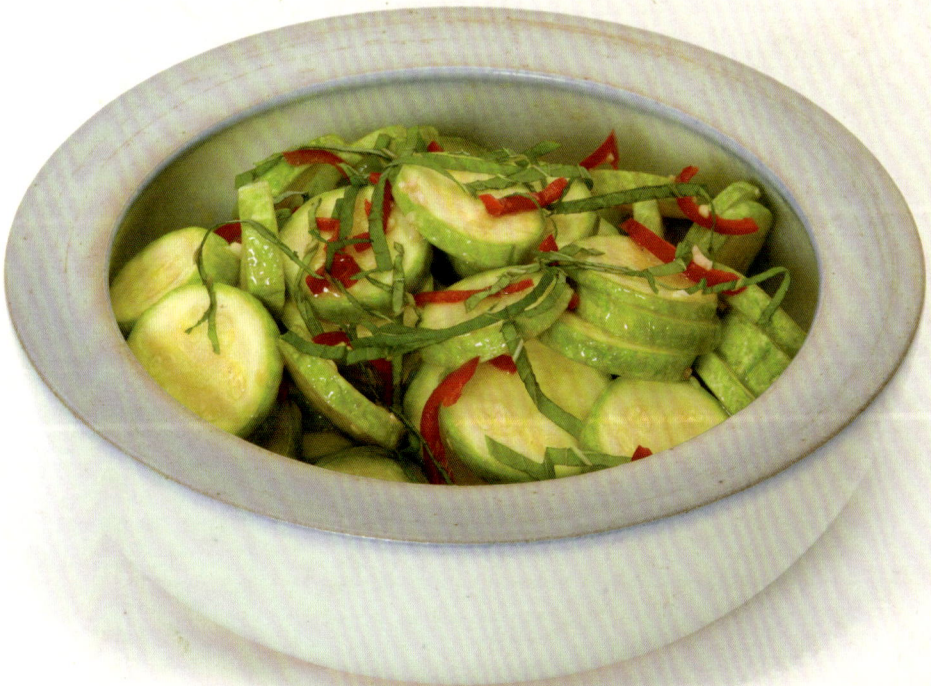

Warm puy lentils with shallot vinaigrette

— SERVES 4 —

Puy lentils used to be an ingredient found only in expensive providores. I'm so very pleased that I can now find them on my supermarket shelves with their lovely speckled colour and, when cooked, that nutty sweetness. Puy style lentils tend to keep their shape and texture when cooked and I find them to be not only delicious but so beautiful to the eye.

300 grams (10.5 ounces) of dried puy style lentils

One large bouquet garni of thyme, parsley stalks and bay leaves

One onion studded with two cloves

1 whole garlic clove unpeeled

1.5 litres (6 cups) of cold water

VINAIGRETTE

2 teaspoons of Dijon mustard

60mL (¼ cup) of white wine vinegar

1 clove of garlic crushed

6 shallots (eschallots) finely chopped

125mL (½ cup) of walnut oil

Salt and pepper

2 tablespoons of parsley finely chopped

1. Place the lentils, bouquet garni, onion studded with cloves and whole garlic clove into a large saucepan and pour over the cold water.

2. Place the covered pan over a high heat and bring it to the boil. Reduce the heat to low so a steady simmer is maintained until the lentils have become tender. This will take around 20 minutes depending on the age of the lentils. While the lentils are simmering you can prepare the vinaigrette.

3. Into a medium sized bowl add the mustard, vinegar, garlic and shallots and whisk them together. Slowly drizzle the walnut oil into the vinegar whisking continuously so it emulsifies into the vinaigrette. Be liberal with the salt and freshly ground pepper as you have not seasoned the lentils at all.

4. Once the lentils are cooked remove the bouquet garni, onion and garlic and drain thoroughly.

5. Pour over the shallot vinaigrette and stir gently so every single lentil is coated in the wonderful vinaigrette. Set the lentils aside for five minutes to allow the vinaigrette to start to absorb into the lentils.

6. Just before serving stir through the parsley and do a final check of the seasoning.

Desserts

EATING OUT has become easier with many cafes and restaurants now identifying dishes as gluten free by displaying a 'GF' on the menu. Pizzerias now offer gluten free pizza bases, Asian restaurants will use tamari rather than soy sauce containing wheat and I haven't seen a café breakfast menu that doesn't offer gluten free bread in years.

If you are dining at a restaurant and they have not identified any gluten free options on their menu just have a word with your waiter and they will be able to make some recommendations. The chef can also adjust most dishes to cater to your dietary needs — this might be as simple as the exclusion of a pre-prepared flour thickened sauce or replacing a biscuit crumb with a scattering of toasted nuts.

When booking a table let the restaurant know of your dietary requirements so they can plan for your needs. I have dined in some restaurants where they have provided me with a full menu containing only gluten free options. This is a wonderful approach and has made me feel so free when selecting my dishes.

The important thing to note when dining out is that you have to be confident that your dietary requirements are understood and are able to be catered for — if you have doubts it's much better to ask questions, or in the extreme case choose to dine elsewhere rather than risk your health.

I have not had one of these experiences for a couple of years thanks to the education that has occurred across the industry.

Chefs are also starting to learn and think about gluten free alternatives to their standard recipes. This includes simple things such as using gluten free flours to thicken sauces. The explosion of quinoa on restaurant and café menus over recent years is another example of the power that dietary needs have had on the industry. Not only is quinoa a fantastically healthy option, it has a great texture and is incredibly versatile as it takes on the flavours of the other ingredients.

There is one section of the menu that I feel chefs still have much to learn about: desserts.

There are generally one or two gluten free options but the usual suspects appear again and again: flourless orange and almond cake, flourless chocolate cake, raspberry friand, a meringue or maybe a scoop of ice-cream or sorbet.

Now these are all beautiful and delicious desserts but it's such a shame that more adventurous options aren't available. There are so many wonderful desserts that can easily be converted to gluten free, so hopefully we will start to see this trend on restaurant menus over the coming months and years.

Apricot and sauvignon blanc jellies

— SERVES 6 —

This recipe will make four individually sized serves to form a delicate end to a dinner party. I have served these in espresso glasses as part of a dessert course at a large party with guests standing around enjoying their jelly with teaspoons. It is beautiful topped with fresh raspberries.

1 kilogram (2.2 pounds) of ripe apricots

750mL (3 cups) of sauvignon blanc

200 grams (1 cup) of golden caster sugar

5 leaves of gelatin (2 grams or 0.07 ounces each)

FOR SERVING

Thickened cream

Fresh raspberries

1. Place the apricots into a large saucepan and pour over the sauvignon blanc. Place the pot over a high heat and bring it to the boil. As soon as it boils add the sugar and reduce the heat to maintain a gentle simmer for 20 to 30 minutes or until the fruit have softened and are just holding their shape.

2. Use a slotted spoon to gently remove the fruit from the liquid and set them aside to cool. Taste the liquid and add a little sugar if needed. Once you are happy with the flavour turn off the heat and strain the liquid through a fine strainer into a large measuring jug.

3. Measure the liquid, which will vary depending on how ripe the apricots were and therefore how much of their juice was released during the cooking process.

4. You can adjust the amount of gelatin required based on how much liquid you have.

5. Place the gelatin leaves into a bowl of cold water and allow them to soften for around five minutes before squeezing out the excess liquid and adding them to the sauvignon blanc. Stir the mixture until the gelatin disappears before setting it aside to cool to room temperature.

6. Once the liquid has cooled pour it into four (preferably glass) ramekins and place them in the refrigerator to set.

7. To serve these individual jellies I like to take eight of the stewed apricots and peel them before cutting them into segments and laying them over the top of the set jellies. I then pour some thickened cream in a thin layer over the top of the fruit and finish with a few fresh raspberries.

Steamed golden syrup pudding

— SERVES 6 —

My childhood Sundays usually featured a traditional roast dinner and dessert was always a very traditional English pudding — be it lemon delicious, chocolate self-saucing or a steamed pudding of some description. My mother never made golden syrup pudding when I was a child so this is something I discovered in adulthood. In this recipe I include the warmth of ginger which cuts through the sweetness of the golden syrup.

150 grams (⅔ cup) of unsalted butter softened

170 grams (¾ cup) of golden caster sugar

2 eggs

160 grams (1 cup and 1 tablespoon) of super-fine white rice flour

80 grams (½ cup) of glutinous rice flour

15 grams (4 teaspoons) of gluten free baking powder

2 teaspoons of ground ginger

1 teaspoon of ground nutmeg

85mL (⅓ cup) of milk

125mL (½ cup) of golden syrup

60mL (¼ cup) of golden syrup for serving

1. Grease a 1.2 litre (6 cup) pudding bowl with butter and line the bottom with a circle of baking paper. Set this aside while you prepare the pudding batter.

2. Place the softened butter and sugar into the bowl of your bench-top mixer. With the whisk attachment secured, start at a low speed to roughly incorporate the ingredients before turning to the highest speed setting and allowing it to beat until the mixture is white and fluffy. You may need to stop the mixer occasionally to scrape down the sides.

3. If you don't have a bench-top mixer then you can cream these ingredients by hand with a wooden spoon or with a pair of hand-held rotary beaters.

4. You can check if the mixture is ready by rubbing a small amount between your thumb and forefinger — you shouldn't be able to feel the sugar crystals anymore as they will have dissolved.

5. Once the mixture is ready, add in the eggs one at a time and beat on the highest speed setting until completely incorporated and the mixture has returned to its fluffy texture.

6. Remove the bowl from the mixer and sift the flours, baking powder, ginger and cinnamon. Pour in the milk and use a wooden spoon to combine the ingredients into a smooth batter.

7. Pour the golden syrup into the bottom of your pudding basin and then pour over the pudding batter. Smooth the top of the pudding and then cover with a circle of baking paper. If you have a pudding bowl with a lid secure the lid now otherwise take some aluminium foil and cover the top of the bowl snugly before tying with string to ensure steam does not escape from the bowl while it is steaming. Tie some string across the top of the bowl as well to act as a handle which will make it easier to remove the hot pudding from the pot once it has finished steaming.

8. Fill your kettle and bring it to the boil. Scrunch a piece of aluminium foil into a rough ball — this will act as a trivet for your pudding to stand on to ensure the bottom doesn't burn. Place your handmade trivet into a pot that is tall enough for your pudding bowl to stand with the lid of the pot on.

9. Place the pudding bowl on top of your homemade trivet in the centre of the pot. Pour boiling water into the pot until it is half to two thirds of the way up the side of the pudding bowl.

10. Place the pot over a high heat to bring the water back to the boil before placing the lid on the pot and reducing the heat to low so a gentle simmer is maintained.

11. Steam the pudding for an hour and a half checking and adding more water to the pot if required.

12. Once the pudding has finished steaming, remove the bowl from the pot and remove the foil and baking paper from the top of the pudding bowl. The lovely sweet steam will be released and a beautifully light spongy pudding will be revealed.

13. Invert the pudding bowl onto your serving platter and lift off the bowl. The bottom of the pudding will be golden with the syrup having infused into the sponge.

14. Heat the additional golden syrup in a small saucepan until hot and drizzle this over the top of the pudding just before serving along with some luscious vanilla custard.

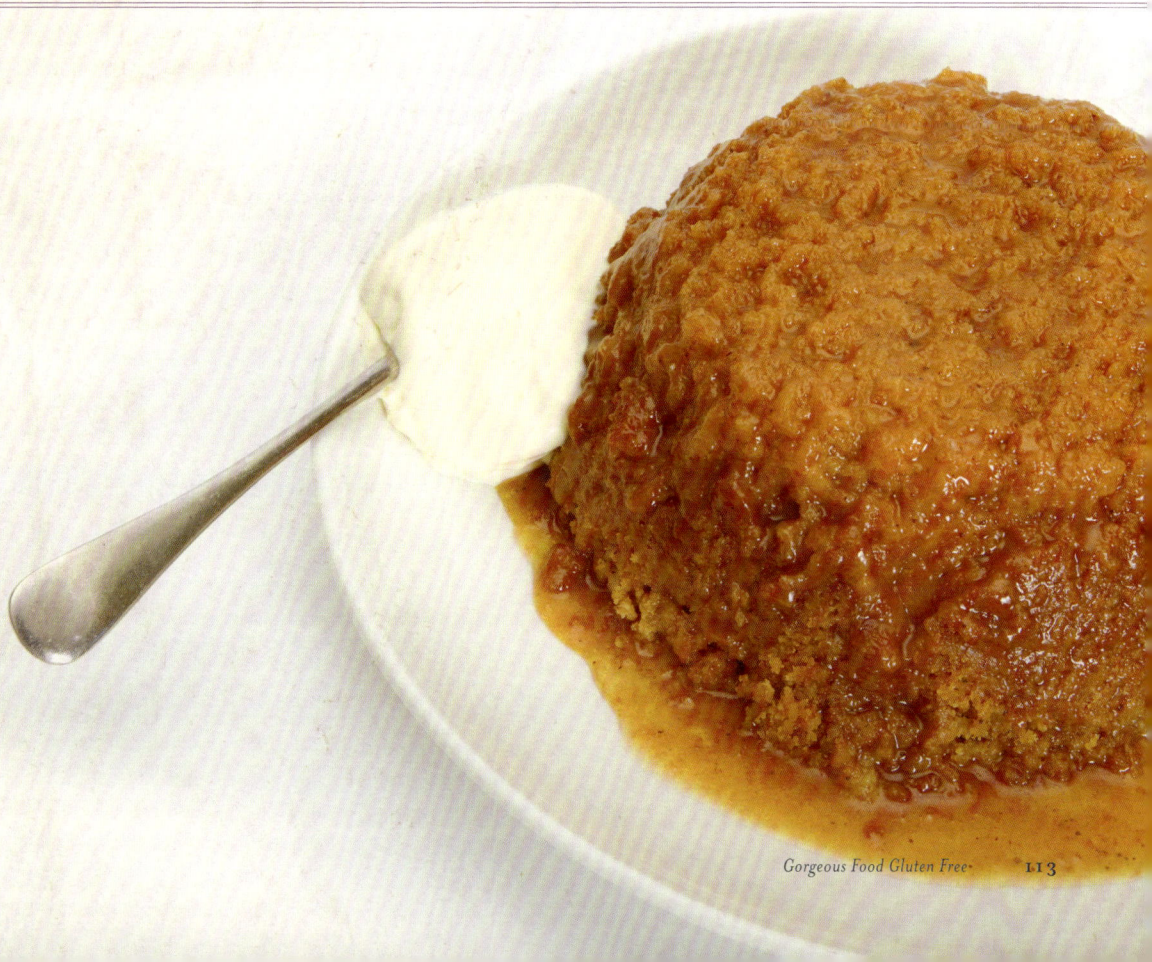

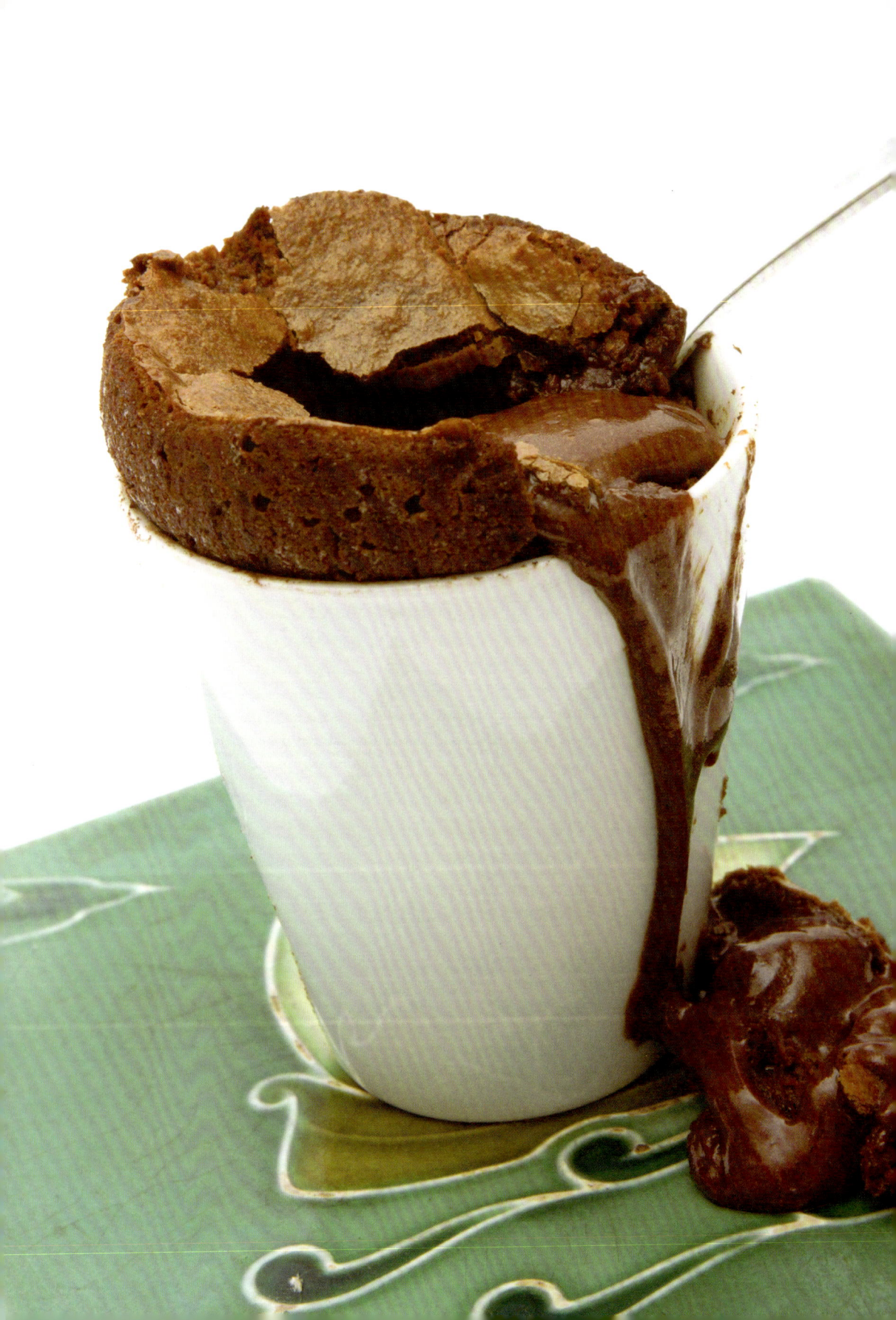

Chocolate fondants

— SERVES 8 —

Fondants often cause a trepidatious weakening of the knees when people consider making a batch. But they create a warm glow around the heart with the mere thought of eating that gooey molten middle. The truth is they are actually very simple to make and this recipe is my take on the cult classic.

40 grams (1.4 ounces) of melted unsalted butter to grease the ramekins

Cocoa to coat the butter-greased ramekins

275 grams (9.7 ounces) the best quality dark chocolate you can afford

225 grams (7.9 ounces) of unsalted butter

300 grams (1⅓ cups) of golden caster sugar

1 teaspoon of vanilla bean paste

5 eggs

140 grams (1 cup) of super-fine white rice flour

60 grams (¼ cup plus 1 tablespoon) of glutinous rice flour

Crème fraiche for serving

1. Take eight ramekins and use a pastry brush to grease the base and sides of each. Brush the butter up the sides of the ramekins as this will help the fondants rise up the grooves left by the brush. Place the ramekins in the refrigerator for a few minutes to allow the butter to set.

2. After the butter has set repeat the process of brushing melted butter up the sides and over the base of the ramekin. Add a teaspoon of cocoa to each ramekin and roll it around to form an even coating over the base and sides. Tip out any excess cocoa and return the ramekins to the refrigerator while you prepare the fondant batter.

3. Pour some water into a medium sized saucepan and bring it to the boil. Turn the heat to low so the water is just simmering and place a metal or ceramic bowl over the saucepan being careful that the base of the bowl does not touch the water.

4. Break the chocolate up into pieces and add these along with the butter to the bowl. Stir the chocolate and butter with a metal spoon until it has melted and then remove the bowl from the heat and take the saucepan off the heat. Set the chocolate and butter mixture aside to cool while you prepare the eggs.

5. Place the eggs, sugar and vanilla bean paste into the bowl of your benchtop mixer. With the whisk attachment secured, start at a low speed to roughly incorporate the ingredients before turning to the highest speed setting and allowing it to beat until the mixture is pale and fluffy and the whisk leaves a trail.

6. If you don't have a bench-top mixer then you can whisk these ingredients by hand with a balloon whisk or with a pair of hand-held rotary beaters.

7. Remove the bowl from the mixer and sift in the flours. Use a large metal spoon to gently fold the flour through the egg mixture being careful to keep as much air as possible in the batter.

8. Pour a third of the cooled chocolate mixture into the batter and again use the large metal spoon to gently fold it through. Repeat this process twice more to incorporate the rest of the chocolate mixture.

9. If your mixing bowl has a pouring lip then you should be able to pour the batter straight into the ramekins. If not I recommend you pour the batter into a jug to make it easier to fill the ramekins.

10. Pour the batter evenly between the eight ramekins and then return them to the refrigerator for at least half an hour. You can keep the fondants at this stage for up to 24 hours so it's a great thing to prepare the day before a dinner party.

11. Place a shelf in the middle of your oven before preheating to a temperature of 200°C/390°F.

12. Place the chilled fondants onto a baking tray and place them into the preheated oven. The fondants will need to cook for 12 minutes and when ready will have a lovely crust on the top and will start to pull away from the side of the ramekins.

13. Remove the fondants from the oven and leave them to sit for a minute before turning them out.

14. Take the first ramekin in your non-preferred hand and use the fingers of your preferred hand to gently pull the edges of the fondant away from the side of the ramekin. Gently tip the fondant slightly onto your preferred hand so you are certain that you have loosened it sufficiently. Gently return the fondant to the ramekin and place the serving plate over the top. Then invert them so the fondant is upside down on the centre of the serving plate.

15. Repeat the process for the remaining fondants before sprinkling them with some extra cocoa and adding a quenelle of crème fraiche to each plate. Serve immediately.

Chocolate roulade filled with cream and fresh berries

— SERVES 6 —

Light sweet chocolate sponge, Chantilly cream and sun-ripened strawberries. This is a crowd-pleaser from the moment the sugar-coated roulade is presented to the table. Once sliced into spiralled rounds and served on individual plates its inner beauty is revealed.

3 eggs separated

125 grams (½ cup) of golden caster sugar

2 tablespoons of cocoa sifted

1 teaspoon of vanilla bean paste

190mL (¾ cup) of thickened (heavy) cream

1 tablespoon of icing sugar

1 punnet of ripe strawberries sliced

1. Place a shelf in the middle of your oven before preheating to a temperature of 180°C/355°F. Line a medium baking tray with baking paper before setting it aside while you prepare the sponge mixture.

2. Place the egg yolks into a large mixing bowl and use a rotary beater to beat them until they turn pale yellow and become thick and creamy. Gradually add the sugar about two tablespoons at a time and bring the mixture back to its creamy texture before adding the next batch of sugar. Once you have incorporated all the sugar sift in the cocoa and beat this through the egg mixture until well incorporated.

3. Place the egg whites into the bowl of your benchtop mixer and whisk them on the highest speed until soft peaks are formed.

4. Take a third of the egg whites and use a large metal spoon to incorporate them into the chocolate mixture. Repeat this process in two more batches until all the egg whites have been folded through and you have a light fluffy mixture.

5. Pour this onto your lined baking tray and smooth the surface before placing it into the preheated oven.

6. Bake the sponge for 15 minutes until the cake has pulled away from the edges of the tin and it springs back when lightly touched in the middle.

7. Sprinkle a clean tea (dish) towel liberally with golden caster sugar and then turn the sponge out onto the sugary surface. Peel away the baking paper and roll up the cake (including the tea towel). Place the roll on a wire rack to cool.

8. Once the sponge has cooled completely whip the cream and fold through the sifted icing sugar.

9. Carefully unroll the cooled sponge and spread the whipped cream in an even layer all the way to the edges of the sponge. Scatter over the sliced strawberries and then use the tea towel to gently re-roll the cake.

10. Carefully pick up the roulade and place it on the serving platter. I like to garnish the platter with a few extra strawberries and some mint leaves.

Lemon tart

— SERVES 8 —

Lemon holds a special place in our home — it is such a versatile fruit and the sharp acidity not only imparts wonderful flavour but also acts in a similar way to salt in that it brings out the flavour of other foods so they taste more of themselves. This recipe for this most perfect of desserts provides creaminess from the crème fraiche but a good amount of lemon ensures the zing that I seek.

PASTRY

130 grams (1 cup) of super-fine white rice flour

70 grams (½ cup) of glutinous rice flour

110 grams (3.9 ounces) of cold unsalted butter, cubed

Pinch of salt

2 to 3 tablespoons of cold water

FILLING

Finely grated zest and juice of five lemons

300mL (1 cup plus 2 tablespoons) of crème fraiche

9 eggs

390 grams (1¾ cup) of white caster sugar

1. Place the flours, butter and salt in the bowl of your food processor and pulse until the mixture resembles bread crumbs. Slowly add the cold water until the dough comes together and forms a ball.

2. Remove the dough from the food processor and roll it out thin between two sheets of baking paper.

3. Gently ease the pastry into a 30cm (11.8 inch) tart pan — the pastry is very soft so any holes can easily be repaired. Once you have an evenly lined pastry shell place the pastry into the refrigerator for at least 30 minutes.

4. While the pastry is chilling place a shelf in the middle of your oven before preheating to a temperature of 190°C/375°F.

5. Remove the tart shell from the refrigerator and line it with a piece of baking paper and pour in some pastry weights or dried beans. Place the tart shell into the oven and bake it for 15 minutes. Remove the pastry weights and return the tart shell to the oven for five minutes before setting it aside to cool while you prepare the filling. Reduce the oven temperature to 120°C/250°F.

6. Pour some water into a medium sized saucepan and bring it to the boil. Turn the heat to low so the water is just simmering and place a metal or ceramic bowl over the saucepan being careful that the base of the bowl does not touch the water.

7. Add all the filling ingredients into the bowl and use a spatula to stir continuously while the sugar dissolves and all the ingredients combine together. Once the mixture reaches a temperature of 60°C/140°F remove the bowl from the heat and pour the mixture through a fine sieve and into the pastry shell. Allow the bubbles to come to the surface and use a spoon to pop them and remove any remaining froth.

8. Place the filled tart into the oven and bake for 25 minutes or until the top has a golden tinge and the filling is set but still has a slight wobble in the centre. You can check that the filling is ready by confirming that it has reached a temperature of 70°C/160°F.

9. Allow the tart to cool completely before serving accompanied by some extra crème fraiche.

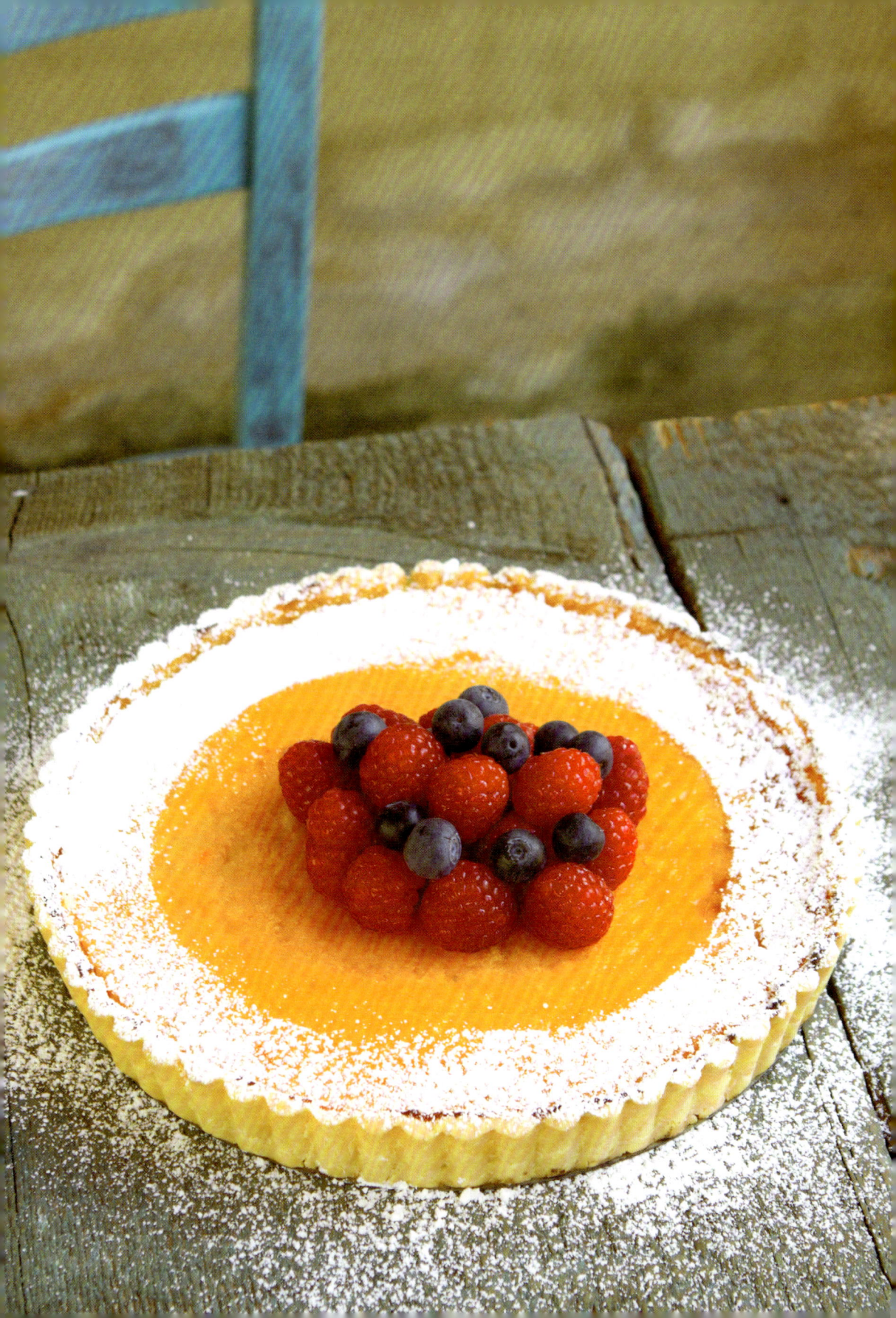

Spiced pear streusel cake

— SERVES 8 —

A traditional streusel cake has a layer of sugary nuts and spices in the centre. In this recipe I take the idea of streusel but instead of adding this layer to the centre of the cake before baking I actually roast the streusel mixture first and then stir this through the cake batter. This gives a wonderful texture to the cake and the pears contribute their lovely sweetness.

STREUSEL

2 teaspoons of ground cinnamon

1 teaspoon of ground nutmeg

1 teaspoon of ground ginger

½ teaspoon of ground cloves

125 grams (½ cup) of unsalted butter softened

260 grams (2⅓ cups) of walnuts roughly chopped

150 grams (¾ cup) of light muscovado sugar

CAKE

150 grams (⅔ cup) of unsalted butter softened

150 grams (⅔ cup) of golden caster sugar

3 eggs

240 grams (1 cup) of sour cream

2 teaspoons of vanilla bean paste

175 grams (1¼ cups) of super-fine white rice flour

90 grams (⅔ cup) of glutinous rice flour

20 grams (4 teaspoons) of gluten free baking powder

3 large ripe pears

1. Place a shelf in the middle of your oven before preheating to a temperature of 170°C/340°F. Grease a 23cm (9 inch) spring-form cake tin with butter and then line the base with grease-proof paper. Also line a baking tray with baking paper.

2. Place all the streusel ingredients into a mixing bowl and use your fingertips to bring it together into a rough paste. Spread this out in a thin, even layer on your lined baking tray and place it in the preheated oven to bake for 15 minutes until it has turned a rich golden colour and the nuts have roasted. Remove the tray from the oven and set it aside while you prepare the cake batter.

3. Place the softened butter and sugar into the bowl of your bench-top mixer. With the whisk attachment secured, start at a low speed to roughly incorporate the ingredients before turning to the highest speed setting and allowing it to beat until the mixture is white and fluffy. You may need to stop the mixer occasionally to scrape down the sides.

4. If you don't have a bench-top mixer then you can cream these ingredients by hand with a wooden spoon or with a pair of hand-held rotary beaters.

5. You can check if the mixture is ready by rubbing a small amount between your thumb and forefinger — you shouldn't be able to feel the sugar crystals any more as they will have dissolved.

6. Once the mixture is ready, add the eggs one at a time, beating until each is completely incorporated and the mixture has returned to its fluffy texture.

7. Add the sour cream and vanilla bean paste and beat until incorporated and the mixture is smooth.

8. Place a sieve over the mixing bowl and sift in the rice flours and baking powder. Gently fold through the dry ingredients with a large metal spoon until combined. Now take the cooled streusel mixture and add this to the cake batter. Don't break it up as it will crumble as you stir it gently through the batter. If you can keep some larger chunks of streusel all the better but don't worry too much about this, just be sure to mix the batter thoroughly.

9. Now peel your pears and cut them in half. Remove the cores and slice them into wedges — depending on the size of the pears you should have around eight slices from each pear.

10. Arrange the pear slices in the bottom of the lined cake tin — the pears will end up on the top of the cake so arrange them in as attractive a manner as you can.

11. Now pour the cake batter over the top of the fruit and smooth the surface.

12. Place the cake in the pre-heated oven and bake for around 35 minutes. You can check if the cake is cooked by placing a wooden skewer into the centre and if it comes out clean then it is ready. It will also have just started to pull away from the sides of the tin.

13. Remove the cake from the oven and leave it to cool for 10 minutes before removing the collar of the spring-form pan. Let the cake cool completely before turning it upside down on the serving platter. Serve this cake with some luscious clotted cream — it doesn't need anything more.

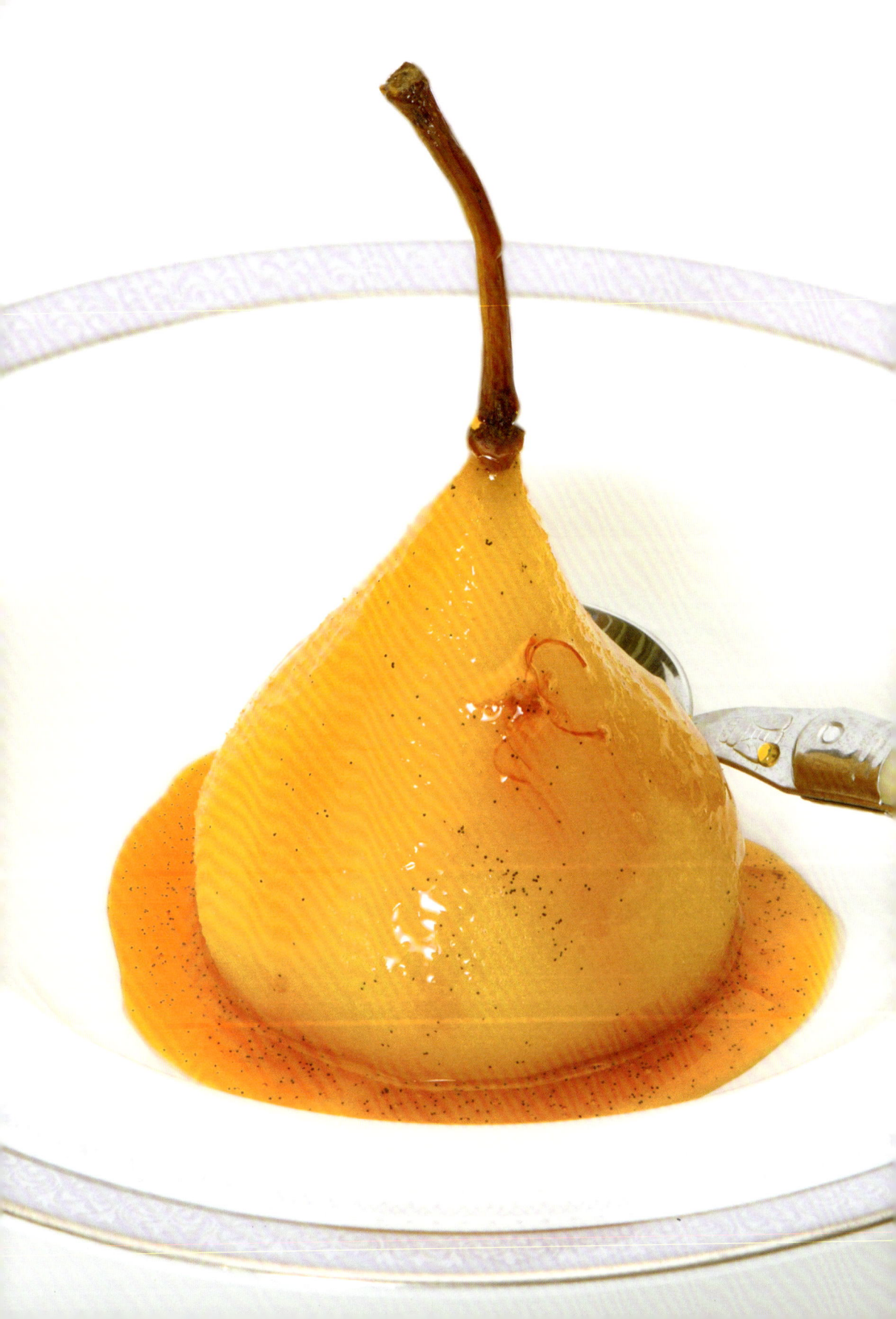

Saffron and vanilla poached pears

— SERVES 4 —

There is something very sensuous about the shape of a perfectly ripe pear. This recipe combines the floral sweetness of vanilla and the earthy depth of saffron to deliver an elegant and sophisticated dessert. You need to have pears that are ripe but still firm — if too soft they will lose their shape as they cook and start to break down.

4 ripe pears

750mL (3 cups) of sauvignon blanc

200 grams (1 cup) of golden caster sugar

2 teaspoons of vanilla bean paste

3 grams of saffron (a large pinch)

FOR SERVING

Thickened cream

1. Boil some water and pour a few tablespoons over the saffron threads and set them aside to steep.

2. Choose pears that have some stem still attached to them and that stand up when placed on their base.

3. Carefully peel your pears and use a melon baller to scoop out the core from the base of each fruit. This allows you to maintain the beauty of the whole fruit while also allowing it to cook from the inside as well as the outside which will result in a more even texture in the final dish.

4. Stand the fruit in a saucepan just large enough for them to fit standing up in the bottom of the pot and with a little space between the fruit. The lid will also need to be able to fit with the fruit standing up.

5. Remove the pears from the saucepan and set them aside while you prepare the stewing liquid.

6. Pour the wine into the saucepan and add the sugar, vanilla bean paste and the water and the saffron water and threads.

7. Place the pan over a high heat and bring it to the boil. Place the pears standing up in the pan and cover with the lid. If the pears are not immersed in the liquid you will need to turn them a few times during the poaching process so they colour evenly in the saffron-scented wine.

8. Once the liquid has returned to the boil reduce the heat to maintain a gentle simmer. Poach the pears for 20 to 30 minutes until the tip of a sharp knife can be easily inserted into the flesh.

9. Gently remove the pears from the poaching liquid and set them aside to cool while you reduce the poaching syrup to form the sauce.

10. Place the saucepan with the poaching syrup over a high heat and bring it to the boil. Allow the syrup to boil vigorously until it has reduced down by two thirds. This will mean you have around one cup (250mL) of golden syrup ready to be drizzled over the pears.

11. To serve place each pear into a shallow bowl and then drizzle the syrup over each pear before pouring over a little cream.

Caramel baked rice pudding

— SERVES 8 —

I was wandering down the Rue de Buci in the 6th arrondissement of Paris one winter afternoon and came across a gorgeous little épicerie full of cheeses and charcuterie, salads, olives and a large baking dish of the most wonderful caramel rice pudding I had ever seen. I bought a large slice and returned triumphantly to our apartment where my husband and I seemingly inhaled our loot in about 5 minutes flat. I don't claim that this recipe can meet the stunning luxury of that Parisian original but this is as close as I can get to the perfection of the rice pudding in my memory.

2 litres (8 cups) of milk

200 grams (1 cup) of short grain white rice

2 vanilla beans split

1 teaspoon of cinnamon

A large pinch of salt

90 grams (scant ½ cup) of golden caster sugar

6 eggs lightly beaten

CARAMEL

200 grams (1 cup) of golden caster sugar

120mL (½ cup) of water

1. Pour the milk into a large saucepan and bring it to the boil. Remove the milk from the heat and scrape in the seeds of the vanilla pods and then add the pods themselves, cinnamon and salt. Return the milk to the heat and bring it back to the boil. Add the rice and continue to stir to ensure the rice doesn't stick together at the bottom of the pan.

2. Once the milk comes back to the boil reduce the heat so the milk is simmering very gently. Let the rice simmer uncovered for around 30 minutes, stirring it occasionally and more frequently as it thickens towards the end of the cooking time. When ready the rice will be very soft but still hold the shape of each individual grain and the milk will have been completely absorbed. The texture should be creamy and when tipped from a spoon should easily slide in luscious splodges back into the pan.

3. Remove the pan from the heat and add the sugar to the creamed rice. Once the sugar has been well incorporated remove the vanilla pods and set the rice aside to cool.

4. Place a shelf in the middle of your oven before preheating to a temperature of 180°C/355°F. while you prepare the caramel.

5. Add the sugar to a medium sized saucepan along with the water and place this over a high heat. To move the sugar around you can shake the pan from time to time but be careful not to slop the mixture over the side of the pan as it will be extremely hot.

6. Bring the sugar to the boil and let it keep boiling until the sugar dissolves and the syrup will then start to colour around the sides of the pan. Reduce the heat and keep shaking and swirling the pan while the syrup turns a deep dark caramel colour. This will take around 5 minutes so be patient and do not leave the caramel alone during this process as it will turn quickly and burn if not closely monitored.

7. Once you have achieved the dark mahogany colour remove the pan from the heat and immediately pour the caramel into the bottom of a large baking dish. I like to use a tempered ovenproof glass dish so you can see the rice and caramel from the side.

8. Tilt the baking dish so you achieve a lovely even caramel layer and leave it to cool for 5 minutes while you finish preparing the rice.

9. Take the now just warm rice and stir through the lightly beaten eggs. Pour this rice custard mixture over the top of the cooled caramel.

10. To ensure the pudding retains its velvety texture the eggs need to cook very gently and evenly. To achieve this, the pudding is baked in a water bath.

11. Fill your kettle with water and bring it to the boil. Place a folded tea (dish) towel in the bottom of a roasting pan that is large enough to hold the pudding dish. Position the pudding in the centre of the roasting pan and then carefully pour boiling water into the side of the roasting pan until it reaches just over half-way up the side of the baking dish.

12. Place the pan into the preheated oven and bake for around 40 minutes or until the pudding has just set in the middle. Remove the baking dish from the water bath and leave the pudding aside to cool.

13. This pudding is best served at room temperature but can be eaten cold from the refrigerator or still slightly warm from the oven. The lovely caramel on the bottom will have largely absorbed into the rice creating a beautiful golden base.

14. Some people like to turn the pudding out in the manner of a crème caramel but personally I prefer to bring the baking dish to the table and use a large metal spoon to scoop out generous portions to reveal the golden secret below.

Notes:

Notes:

Index